10-Minute Tui Na Massage

Text by Liu Naigang
Translation by Shelly Bryant
Cover Design by Shi Hanlin
Interior Design by Wang Wei

Assistant Editors: Qiu Yan, Yang Wenjing
Editor: Cao Yue

ISBN: 978-1-63288-009-3

Address any comments about *10-Minute Tui Na Massage* to:

SCPG
401 Broadway, Ste.1000
New York, NY 10013
USA

or

Shanghai Press and Publishing Development Co., Ltd.
Floor 5, No. 390 Fuzhou Road, Shanghai, China (200001)
Email: sppd@sppdbook.com

Printed in China by Shanghai Donnelley Printing Co., Ltd.

1   3   5   7   9   10   8   6   4   2

10-Minute Tui Na Massage

Natural Healing for **50+** Ailments
through **Traditional Chinese Medicine**

By Liu Naigang

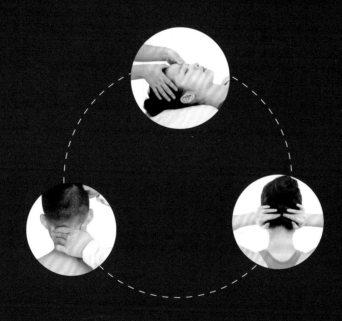

SCPG

TABLE OF CONTENTS

FOREWORD

If you are suffering from a stiff neck but find it a hassle to go to the hospital, how can you alleviate the condition at home using *tui na*?

It is said that menstrual pain can be quickly relieved by massaging the Sanyinjiao acupoint. Is it true?

Is it true that during a *tui na* session, one should work on the area that is causing pain?

What should you do if you cannot locate the acupoint when you are doing self-massage?

This book offers answers to these commonly asked questions.

This book explains the basics of *tui na* in easy-to-understand language and can help beginners pick skills up easily. The book also explains the *tui na* methods to 53 common diseases and 12 *tui na* methods for one's daily wellbeing.

The feature of the book is that it classifies these common diseases and showcases a more targeted *tui na* for the same ailment with different symptoms. The steps are also illustrated in detail to allow beginners with no prior knowledge to pick up *tui na* easily.

This is a healthcare book for home care. Set aside some time every day to do a bit of *tui na* to stimulate the body's immunity, unblock your *qi* and blood, and to stay healthy.

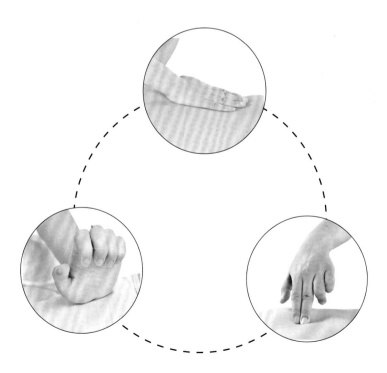

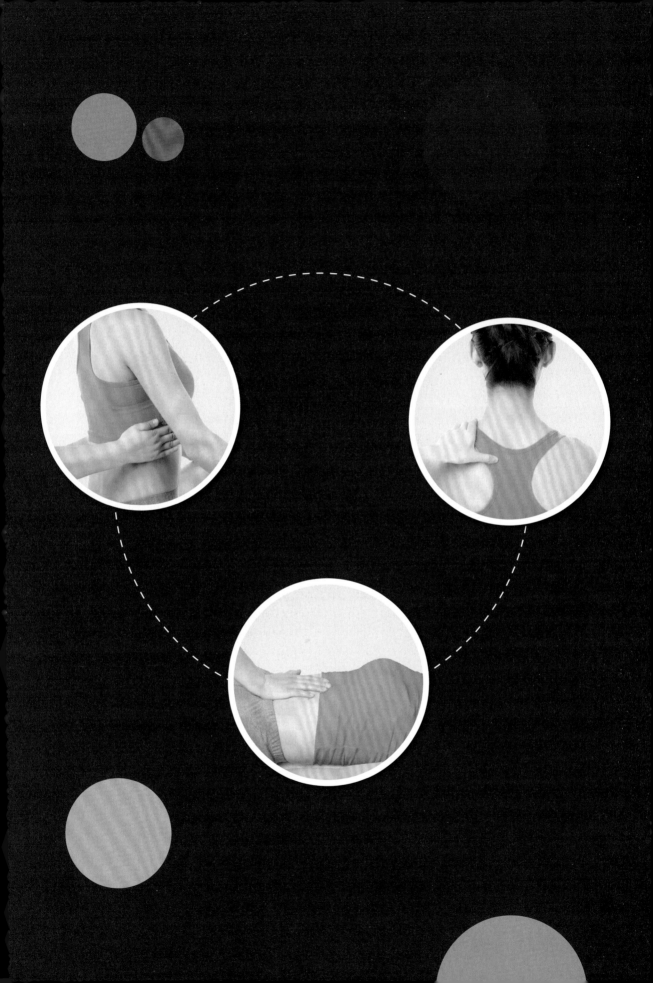

CHAPTER ONE
Basics of *Tui Na*

Traditional Chinese *tui na* is a kind of green therapy which is easy to execute and has few side effects. It is especially suitable for home-based healthcare. This chapter will mainly introduce basic knowledge of *tui na*, such as *tui na* techniques and things to note. This will lay the foundation for subsequent learning.

1. Principles of *Tui Na*

Tui na is the execution of certain techniques on the meridians, acupuncture points, and specific parts on the surface of the human body to adjust its physiological state so as to achieve the purpose of health care and treatment. Why is *tui na* able to maintain health and cure diseases? What effects does *tui na* have on the human body? This can be explained through two principles: the principles of traditional Chinese medicine and the principles of modern medicine.

Principles of Traditional Chinese Medicine

The key to *tui na* is its techniques, which play a crucial role. Standardized, proficient, and appropriate techniques such as the direction of *tui na*, its frequency, strength, stimulation of the affected area, acupoints, and the patient's medical conditions can help regulate the viscera's functions, clear meridians, reconcile *qi* and blood, and heal tendons.

Regulating the viscera's functions: Diseases are developed and formed as a result of the struggle between the body's vital *qi* and pathogenic *qi*. The viscera have the function of receiving and removing turbidity and are responsible for the formation of the *qi* and blood. When the functions of the viscera are off balance, their ability to receive becomes limited, and turbidity becomes difficult to expel, resulting in the weakening of vital *qi* and the accumulation of pathogenic *qi*. By applying the techniques of *tui na* on the corresponding meridians and acupoints on the surface of the human body, functionality of the viscera can be improved, keeping the body in a good state and enhancing one's immunity.

Clearing of meridians: Meridians are the pathways on which *qi* and blood runs in the human body. They have the ability to promote *qi* and blood flow, nourish *yin* and *yang*, and soften the tendons and bones to relieve the joints. When *qi* and blood are not harmonized, external pathogens will invade the meridians and block them, resulting in symptoms such as pain and numbness. *Tui na* can stimulate the surface of the human body to promote the flow of *qi* and blood. The heat generated from *tui na* also accelerates the flow of *qi* and blood, preventing *qi* stagnation and blood stasis, which clears up the meridians.

Reconciling *qi* and blood: Nutrient and defensive *qi* and blood can run through the body and penetrate into the viscera and muscles, harmonizing the human body. When nutrients and defensive *qi* and blood are in tandem, the body is nourished by it and the body is in a harmonized state with balanced *yin* and *yang*. *Tui na* adopts different techniques based on the situation, to apply gentle force on the acupoints to regulate the meridians in order to achieve reconciliation of nutrient and defensive *qi* and keep the body healthy.

Healing tendons: Damage to tendons, bones, and joints can result in collateral damage to the meridians, causing stagnation of *qi* and blood stasis. This causes swelling and pain, affecting limb and joints mobility. Applying *tui na* on the meridians can help the muscles relax. It also disperses the stagnation of *qi* and reduces swelling, eventually healing the injured area. This is specifically reflected in three aspects. First, *tui na* on the injured area helps to promote circulation of *qi* and blood, in turn reducing swelling, regulating *qi*, and relieving pain. Next, *tui na* can adjust and restore tendons by applying force to realign tendons and fix dislocations. Third, appropriate passive techniques can help loosen adhesions and smoothen joints.

Principles of Modern Medicine

Tui na seems to be a form of mechanical stimulation, but skillful and proficient execution of the techniques can produce *gong*. This *gong* has some healing functions and can convert to other energy to work on the systems in the human body, such as nervous, circulatory, digestive, and endocrine, treating different types of ailments.

Regulating the nervous system: *Tui na* has a certain regulatory effect on the nervous system. Its techniques can stimulate the excitatory and inhibitory processes of the central nervous system through a reflex conduction pathway. Studies have shown that stimulation of the Hegu and Zusanli acupoints of a healthy person enhances the α waves in an electroencephalogram (EEG). This indicates that applying stronger force on the meridian during *tui na* can inhibit the cerebral cortex, while applying gentler force on the neck can enhance the α waves of the test subject's EEG, showing that the stimulation of acupoints is the same regardless of the force applied. A patient with insomnia often falls asleep during *tui na* treatment, while a sleepy patient usually becomes refreshed and energetic. This shows that *tui na* has a two-way regulatory effect on the central nervous system.

The stimulation sites and treatment points of the various *tui na* techniques are mostly distributed around the roots, trunks, segments, and passages of the peripheral nerves. The stimulation from *tui na* can improve nerve functions and its conduction pathway, stimulating the peripheral nerves to accelerate their conduction reflexes. At the same time, *tui na* can also improve local blood circulation and nerve nutrition, promoting the recovery of nerve cells and fibers.

Promoting blood circulation: While *tui na* is executed on the body's surface, the pressure applied is transmitted to the walls of blood vessels, prompting blocked blood to suddenly flow again, increasing the strength and speed of blood flow. The rhythmic stimulation of *tui na* can also increase blood flow rate, thereby reducing blood viscosity and prompting the blood a positive correlation cycle between blood flow and blood viscosity. In short, *tui na* can relax muscles and improve the hypercoagulable and hyper-viscosity state of the blood. It also helps to accelerate blood circulation and improve microcirculation and cerebral circulation, alleviating the effects of illnesses such as hypertension, coronary heart disease, and atherosclerosis.

Regulating gastrointestinal function: The direct pressure from *tui na* can help promote morphological change in the gastrointestinal tract. This promotes the movement of bowels and accelerates the speed of gastrointestinal motility, thereby changing the rate of bowel excretion. The stimulation from *tui na* can enhance gastrointestinal motility and bowel excretion through reflex conduction. This in turn promotes the digestion and absorption of food by the stomach and intestines, strengthening the function of the digestive system.

Regulating endocrine: When their Pishu, Geshu, and Zusanli acupoints are massaged, and their Taiyang Bladder Meridian of Foot (one of the twelve main meridians of the human body) are rubbed, some patients with diabetes see an improvement in their pancreatic function, varying degrees of drops in their blood sugar level, a negative result in their urine sugar test, and an improvement in their condition of "drinking more, eating more, diuretics, and weight loss." Applying single finger meditation pushing technique on a patient with hyperthyroidism can help lower their heart rate significantly and improve their other symptoms too.

Relieving muscle fatigue: *Tui na* directly inhibits muscle spasms through muscle stretching reflexes, indirectly relieving muscle tension by elimination the source of the pain. It also relaxes the limbs, eliminates excessive tension and stiffness of skeletal muscles, ensures muscle elasticity, prevents muscle fatigue, and promotes physical recovery.

Easing and relieving pain: *Tui na* can relax soft tissues, improve blood circulation, and promote the dilution, decomposition, and removal of peripheral pain-causing substances, giving it a better pain-relieving effect. The stimulation from *tui na* can inhibit the transmission of pain signals to achieve pain relief. This is helpful in pain caused by strain, physical exercise, and many other chronic pain-inducing ailments. Gentle *tui na* can relieve pain and improve one's mood.

2. Commonly Used *Tui Na* Techniques

There are many types of traditional Chinese medicine *tui na* techniques. Some have the same name but different execution methods, and some have different names but same execution methods. Some are classified based on movement, some are classified based on the requirements of the respective methods, and some are classified based on how they are executed. For easy mastery and application, this book introduces commonly used *tui na* techniques and their requirements for execution. (Note: In the specific steps, if clockwise or anti-clockwise is listed, please follow the instructions accordingly. Otherwise, either direction is acceptable.)

Basic Techniques

① **Rolling Method**

How it works: Place the joint of the pinky back down on the treatment site. Using the flexing motion of the wrist joint and the rotating motion of the forearm, roll the hypothenar and the back of the palm continuously back and forth on the treatment site.

Points to note: Keep shoulders and arms relaxed as much as possible, and keep elbow slightly bent.

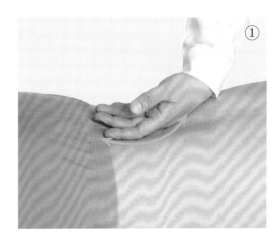

Effect: This method has high pressure and a large contact area. It is suitable for more muscular areas such as shoulders, waist, hips, and limbs. This technique has the effect of relaxing tendons, activating blood circulation, soothing joints, and relieving muscle and ligament spasms.

② Single Finger Meditation Pushing Method

How it works: Apply pressure to the treatment site or acupoint with the tip of the thumb finger, the thumb pulp or the side of the thumb respectively. Relax the wrist, sink the shoulder, droop the elbow, and hang the wrist. The elbow joint should be slightly lower than the wrist. Using the elbow as the fulcrum, move the forearm and allow the wrist and thumb to flex and extend in tandem with the forearm's movement.

    Points to note: When the wrist moves, the ulnar side (pinkie side) of the wrist should be lower than the radial side (thumb side), so that the pressure generated can continue to act on the treatment side. The pressure, frequency, and range of movement should be uniform, but the movement can be flexible.

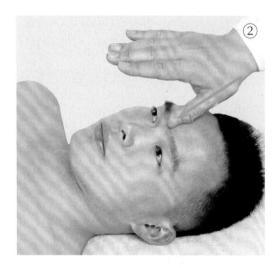

    Effect: This method has a small contact area, but its penetration is high. It is suitable to be used on the whole body and has the effect of relaxing tendons and activating collaterals, regulating the nutrient and defensive *qi*, and dispelling bruises.

③ Kneading Method

Palm kneading method: Using the thenar region or the heel of the palm, place it on the treatment site and exert pressure. Keep the wrist relaxed and use the elbow as the fulcrum. Move the forearm and let the wrist move gently in tandem with the forearm's movement to create a light kneading motion.

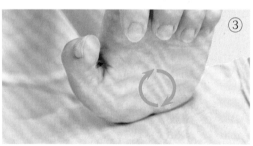

    Finger kneading method: Place the fingertips on the treatment site and exert pressure. Keep the wrist relaxed and use the elbow as the fulcrum. Move the forearm and let the wrist and fingers move gently in tandem with the forearm's movement to create a light kneading motion.

    Points to note: The pressure should be light, and the movement should be coordinated and rhythmic.

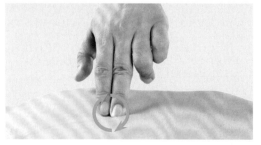

    Effect: This method is gentle and soothing with little stimulation. It is suitable to be used on the whole body. This method has the effect of expanding the lungs and regulating *qi*, promoting blood circulation, and dispelling bruises.

④ Circular Rubbing Method

Palm rubbing method: Place the surface of the palm onto the treatment site. Using the wrist as the center point, perform a rhythmic circular motion by moving the forearm simultaneously.

Finger rubbing method: Close the index finger, middle finger, and ring finger together. Place these fingers onto the treatment site. Using the wrist as the center point, perform a rhythmic circular motion by moving the forearm simultaneously.

Points to note: Allow the elbow to bend naturally and keep the wrist relaxed. Straighten the fingers and palm naturally and take note that the movement should be slow and coordinated.

Effect: This method is gentle and soothing. It is suitable for chest, abdomen, and ribs. This method helps to regulate *qi* of the spleen and stomach, and promote digestion and remove food retention.

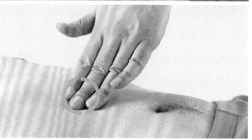

⑤ Pushing Method

How it works: Place fingers, palm, or elbow onto the treatment site and move in a single direction in a straight line. This technique can be called finger pushing, palm pushing, or elbow pushing method, depending on what is used for this *tui na* technique.

Points to note: The fingers, palm, or elbow must be pressed closely to the treatment site. The speed of this technique should be slow and even.

Effect: This method is suitable to be used on the whole body. It helps to relax muscles and activate collaterals.

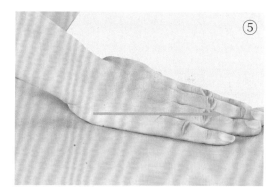

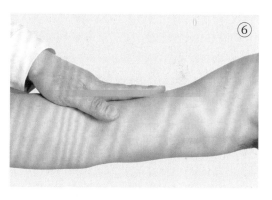

⑥ To-and-Fro Rubbing Method

How it works: Place thenar region, hypothenar or the heel of the palm on the treatment site. Push and rub back and forth in a linear motion. During the execution of this method, the wrist joint should be straightened so that the forearm can be lowered close to the level of the hand. The fingers should also be stretched out naturally, and the whole palm should be placed on the treatment site. The shoulder joint acts as the fulcrum for this technique, and the upper arm is the driver of the movement, pushing and pulling the palm back and forth, or up and down.

Points to note: The force applied should be steady, and the movement should be even and continuous.

Effect: This method provides a warm, gentle stimulation and has the effect of warming the meridians, dredging collaterals, promoting *qi* and blood circulation, reducing swelling, and relieving pain.

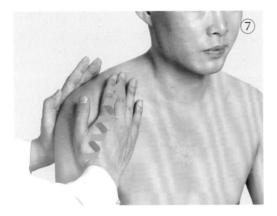

⑦ Palm Twisting Method

How it works: Clamp the treatment site with both palms and rub it quickly with slight force, moving up and down at the same time.

Points to note: The force applied by both hands should be the same. The rubbing should be fast, but the movement up and down should be slow.

Effect: This method is suitable for the lower back, chest, and limbs. It is commonly applied on the upper limbs. This method has the effect of regulating *qi* and blood, relieving muscle rigidity, and activating collaterals.

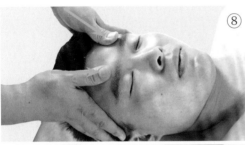

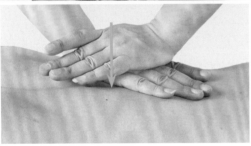

⑧ Pressing Method

Finger pressing method: Press the treatment site with the tip or the pulp of the thumb.

Palm pressing method: This method can be executed with either one or two palms. When using both palms, one can be placed on the other to press on the treatment site.

Points to note: The source of pressure must be placed firmly on the treatment site. The pressure applied should start light and increase progressively.

Effect: The finger pressing method is suitable for the whole body, while the palm pressing method is commonly used on the lower back and abdomen. This method has the effect of relaxing muscles, dredging meridians, promoting blood circulation, and relieving pain.

⑨ Finger Pressing Method

Thumb pressing method: Use the tip of the thumb to press the treatment site.

Finger joint pressing method: Bend the thumb and use the side of the thumb joint to press the treatment site. Alternatively, bend the index finger and use the side of the finger joint to press the treatment site.

Points to note: The difference between the finger pressing and pressing methods is that finger pressing has a smaller area of contact, but it exerts a greater stimulation.

Effect: This method creates strong stimulation, and the force applied should be based on the patient's condition and the location of the treatment site. It is usually used on areas where the muscle is thinner and around bone sutures. This method has the effect of unblocking blockages, promoting blood circulation, relieving pain, and regulating visceral functions.

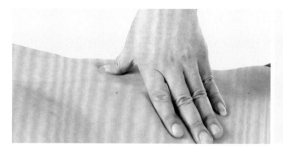

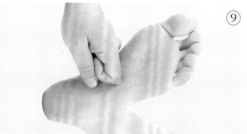

⑩ Pinching Method

Three-finger pinch: Clamp the treatment site with the thumb, index finger, and middle finger. Squeeze with force.

Five-finger pinch: Clamp the treatment site with the thumb and all four fingers. Squeeze with force. When squeezing, the force applied should be even, and the squeezing should be rhythmic.

Points to note: The wrist should be braced when exerting force. When pinching, the finger joints should be kept relaxed, and the pinching should be light and continuous.

Effect: This method is suitable for the head, neck, limbs, and back. This method has the effect of relaxing muscles, activating collaterals, and promoting *qi* and blood circulation.

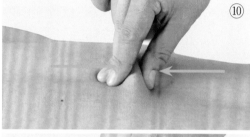

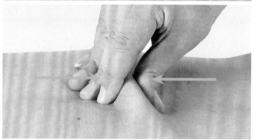

⑪ Grasping Method

How it works: Grasp the treatment site with the thumb, index finger, and middle finger, or the thumb and all four other fingers with light force, and execute a rhythmic grasp-and-lift motion.

Points to note: Start off with light grasping, and slowly apply more force through the course of this method. The motion should be slow and coherent.

Effect: This method is often used in conjunction with other *tui na* methods. It

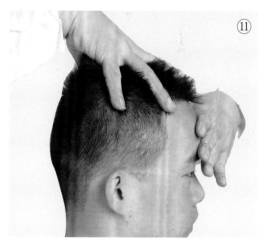

is suitable for the head, neck, shoulders, and limbs. This method has the effect of expelling wind and cold, unblocking acupoints for pain alleviation, relaxing muscles, and activating collaterals.

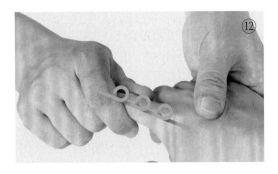

⑫ Holding Twisting Method

How it works: Pinch the treatment site with the thumb and index finger. Perform a knead and twist motion.

Points to note: The movement should be nimble and fast.

Effect: This method is suitable for small joints on the limbs. It has the effect of regulating tendons, activating collaterals, and improving joint mobility.

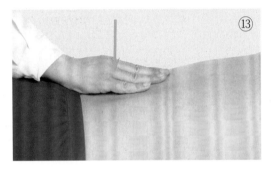

⑬ Patting Method

How it works: Use the hollow of the palm to pat the surface of the treatment site.

Points to note: The fingers should be kept close together naturally, and slightly bent. The patting motion should be steady and rhythmic.

Effect: This method is suitable for the shoulders, back, waist, hips, and lower limbs. It is often used with other *tui na* methods, and can help to relax tendons, activate collaterals, and promote *qi* and blood circulation.

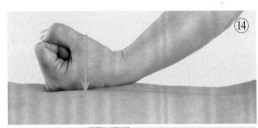

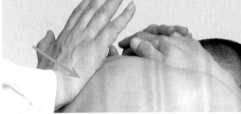

⑭ Striking Method

Fist striking: Clench the palm into a fist and straighten the wrist. Hit the treatment site with the back of the fist.

Palm striking: Keep the fingers open naturally, and straighten the wrist. Strike the treatment area using the heel of the palm.

Side striking: Straighten the fingers naturally, and flex the wrist backwards slightly. Hit the treatment site using the hypothenar of the palm(s).

Fingertip striking: Strike the treatment site using the fingertip, like raindrops.

Points to note: The force applied should be short and quick. The direction of the strike should be vertical towards the body, and there should be no dragging motion. The speed of the strikes should be even and rhythmic.

Effect: Fist striking is commonly used on the lower back; palm striking is often used

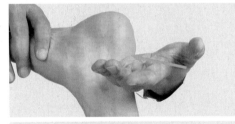

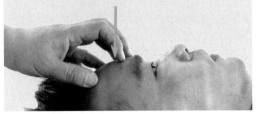

on the top of the head, waist, hip and four limbs; palm side striking is commonly used on the back and the limbs, and fingertip strikes are used on the head, face, chest, and abdomen. This method has the effect of relaxing tendons, activating collaterals, and regulating *qi* and blood.

⑮ Poking Method

How it works: Straighten the thumb and apply force to the treatment site using the tip of the thumb. Place the other four fingers in a corresponding position for support. Press the thumb downwards until the site is sore. Keeping the direction of force applied perpendicular to the muscle fiber (or tendon, ligament), gently shake the thumb back and forth.

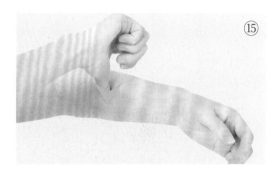

    Points to note: The strength of the force applied should gradually increase, and it should be a firm press. The direction of the force applied should be perpendicular to the tissue of the treatment site.

    Effect: This method has the effect of relieving pain and releasing adhesions.

⑯ Shaking Method

How it works: Hold the patient's wrist or ankle to be treated with both hands and raise it to an angle. Apply force from the forearms and move the hands up and down while shaking them. The vibration generated from the shaking motion is transmitted to the shaken limb, soothing the limb and joint in the process.

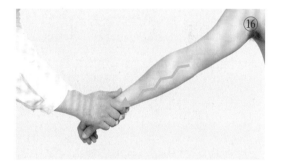

    Points to note: Keep the vibration small but the shaking frequency high.

    Effect: This method can be used on the limbs, particularly the upper limbs. It is commonly used in conjunction with the palm twisting method and is commonly used as the final technique of a *tui na* treatment. This method has the effect of regulating *qi* and blood, relaxing tendons, and activating collaterals.

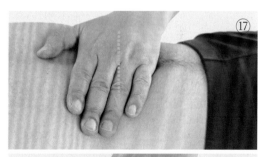

⑰ Vibrating Method

Palm vibrating method: Place the palm firmly on the treatment site and apply force. Keep the forearm and hand muscles tense and make a vibrating motion.

    Finger vibrating method: Place the tip of the middle finger on the treatment site and apply force. Keep the forearm and hand muscles tense and make a vibrating motion.

    Points to note: During the execution

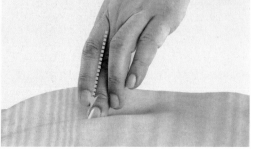

of this method, the force applied should be concentrated on either the palm or the tip of the finger. The force applied should increase in conjunction with the frequency of the vibrations.

Effect: This method can be used on all parts of the body. It has the effects of removing blood stasis, harmonizing *qi* of the spleen and stomach, aiding digestion, and regulating intestinal functions.

⑱ Nipping Method

How it works: Bend the thumb slightly, and pinch and press on the acupoints on the treatment site using the thumb nail.

Points to note: Pinch and press the acupoint with the thumb nail. Apply more force

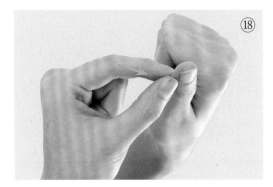

as the area of stimulation is small. To avoid abrasions, it is not advisable to dig the nail into the skin.

Effect: This method has the effect of dredging meridians for *qi* and blood circulation. It is suitable for acupoints on the face and the limbs. It has a strong stimulating effect and helps with unblocking acupoints for spasm relief. This method is often followed by the kneading method to ease the stimulation.

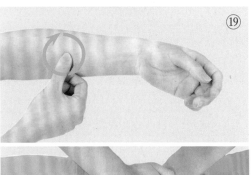

⑲ Pressing-Kneading Method

Pressing-kneading with fingers: Place the thumb on the treatment site with the rest of the fingers on the opposite or corresponding position to assist. Actively apply force with the thumb and forearm, and perform rhythmic compression and kneading.

Pressing-kneading with the palm: Press the heel of the palm of one hand or both hands on the treatment site. Keep the fingers naturally straight. Using the force from the forearm and upper arm, knead and press in a rhythmic motion.

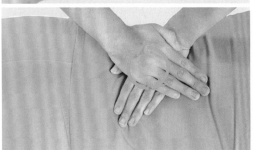

Points to note: This technique is a combination of pressing and kneading methods. It is advisable to press and knead simultaneously. Do not move too fast or too slow.

Effect: Pressing-kneading with fingers covers a small contact area and exerts concentrated force. This method is suitable for the whole body, but especially the neck, shoulders, and inner edge of the scapula. Pressing-kneading with the palm covers a large contact area, and the kneading force is more dispersed.

⑳ Grasping-Kneading Method

How it works: This is a combination of grasping and kneading methods, in which the kneading motion is added when the grasping method is used. When applying the pinching and lifting, add a moderate rotation and kneading motion using the thumb and the other fingers, so that the force is continuously applied to the treatment site.

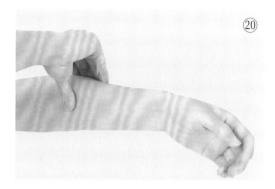

Points to note: Grasping is still the main method here, supplemented by a kneading motion. This method should be executed in a smooth and natural manner.

Effect: The force of this *tui na* method is more moderate than that of the grasping method, and is more natural and comfortable. This method is usually used on the four limbs and neck.

㉑ Kneading-Pinching Method

How it works: On the basis of the pinching method, incorporate a kneading motion using the fingers. The kneading motion of the thumb or heel of the palm should be kept small, while the other fingers continue with the pinching, spiralling forward while kneading and pinching.

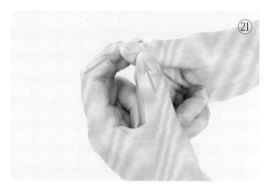

Points to note: Keep the shoulders and elbows relaxed. The fingers should be placed firmly on the treatment site. The force applied should be continuous, even, coordinated, and rhythmic. The strength and frequency of the force applied should be as strong as the patient can tolerate.

Effect: It is suitable for the whole body, especially the neck, four limbs, and local pain conditions.

㉒ Plucking Method

How it works: Apply pressure to the treatment site with the tip of the thumb. When there is local soreness and swelling, make short plucking motions perpendicular to the muscle fibers.

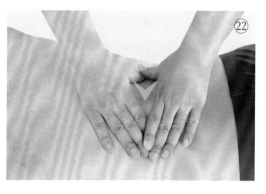

Points to note: The pressure exerted by the fingers should be strong and within the patient's tolerance. The plucking movements should be kept small, so that the deep tissues can produce mutual mis-shift between the motions.

Effect: This is one of the methods that offers stronger stimulation. It has the effects of relaxing tendons and activating joints, breaking down adhesions, and relieving spasms and pain.

㉓ Pushing-Rubbing Method

How it works: Apply pressure to the treatment site with the radial side of the thumb. Keep the other four fingers close together, and apply force on the treatment site. Use the forearm as the main motion driver, and drive the wrist joint in a circular rotation movement. And drive the metacarpophalangeal joint and interphalangeal joint of the thumb to flex and extend, and rub the surface of the other four fingers in a circular motion on the treatment site.

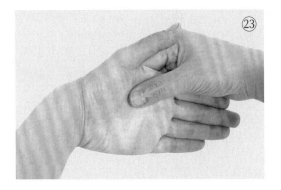

Points to note: The thumb should be placed firmly on the treatment site, and the wrist joints should be relaxed.

Effect: This method is usually used on the chest, abdomen and four limbs. It has the effects of freeing up the lungs and relieving asthma, harmonizing *qi* of spleen and stomach, relaxing tendons and meridians, activating blood, and regulating menstruation.

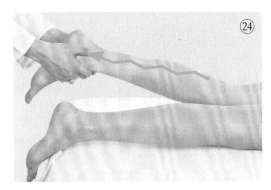

㉔ Pulling-Shaking Method

How it works: Pull and shake the patient's body, particularly at the waist. Have the patient lie down in a prone position and grab the end of the bed with both hands. Then, hold the upper part of the patient's ankles. Pull downwards with force, then relax and swing left and right a few times. When the patient's waist muscles are relaxed, shake 3 to 4 times before repeating the pulling motion.

Points to note: Gaining traction is the first step. Next, reduce the traction before making a larger shaking motion. Pace the timing of the shaking.

Effect: This method is mainly used on the waist, shoulders, and hip joints. It has the effects of smoothening joints, and resetting and loosening adhesions, the instantaneous force is strong.

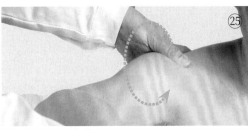

㉕ Rotating Method

Shoulder joint rotation: The patient should be seated. Hold their shoulder with one hand, and their wrist or elbow with the other hand. Shake the shoulder joint to make a clockwise or anti-clockwise rotation.

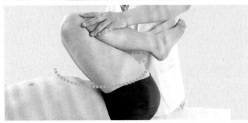

Waist rotation: Have the patient go into a supine position and keep their legs together with the hips and knees flexed. Press both knees with both hands, or press the knee with one hand and the ankle with the other hand. Coordinate the force exerted

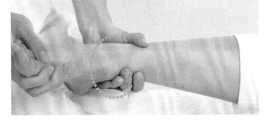

by both arms, and rotate.

Ankle rotation: Have the patient go into a supine position. Hold their heel with one hand, and their ankle joint with the other. Rotate the ankle joint clockwise and anti-clockwise.

Points to note: Make the joints rotate passively. The rotation should go from slow to fast, and the speed should increase progressively. Half of the rotations should be clockwise, and the other half should be anti-clockwise.

Effect: The focus of this method is on joint movement. It is suitable for all joints on the limbs, neck, shoulder, and waist.

㉖ **Pulling Method**

Neck side pulling: With the patient's head bent forward slightly, place one hand on the back of their head and the other on their chin. When the patient rotates their head all the way to the side, tug both hands simultaneously in the opposite direction of the force.

Waist side pulling: Have the patient lie down on their side. Place one hand on the front of their shoulder and the other on their hip. Or place one hand on the back of their shoulder and the other on the anterior superior iliac spine. After passive rotation of the patient's waist to its maximum extent, tug both hands simultaneously in the opposite direction of the force.

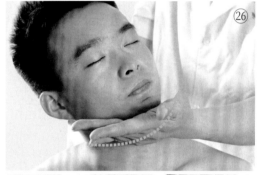
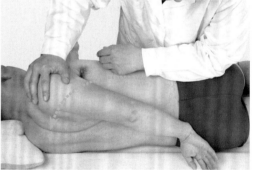

Points to note: This method exerts sudden force on the joints to rotate, flex, and stretch. The method must be executed in a swift and decisive manner and the force exerted should be steady. Both hands must be coordinated, and the pulling must not exceed the physiological range of movement of the joint. The method should be executed in a light and accurate manner.

Effect: This method is commonly used for joint dislocation and joint dysfunction. It has the effects of relaxing the tendons, dredging the collaterals, and lubricating the joints.

㉗ **Stretching Method**

Neck stretching: Have the patient seated. Stand behind them, support the back of their head with one hand and hold their lower jaw with the elbow bent. Support the side of the patient's head with the palm. Pull their head upwards with both hands simultaneously to stretch the cervical vertebrae.

Finger joint stretching: Use one hand to pinch the proximal end of the joint to be pulled and stretched and the other hand to hold the distal end. Pull both hands simultaneously in opposite directions.

Points to note: Secure and steady one end of the body, limb or joint to be pulled, and stretch and pull the other end. The force applied should be even and persistent, and the movement should be gentle.

Effect: This method is commonly used for joint misalignment and tendon injury. It is useful for the rehabilitation of twisted tendons and displaced joints.

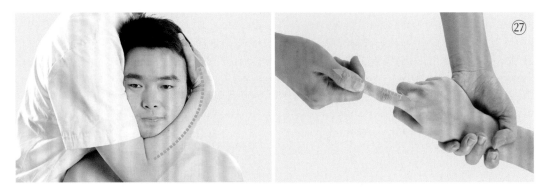

3. Preparation Work before *Tui Na*

In order to achieve the desired therapeutic effect of *tui na*, the following preparations are required before a session.

Before *tui na*, first wash your hands and keep your fingers clean and warm. Nails should be trimmed and blunt, and objects that may hinder the massage (e.g., rings) must be removed so as not to damage the patient's skin. The temperature of the room should be kept comfortable, optimally between 20–25°C to prevent the patient from catching a cold and falling sick.

Posture for *Tui Na*

Having the correct posture helps with the mastery of strength, rhythm, and point of force. This makes the patient more comfortable, and a better outcome can be achieved from the *tui na* session.

Sitting: Sit upright with the knees and hips bent at 90°. The feet should be shoulder-width apart. The arms should droop naturally at the side of the body, and the hands should be placed on the knees. This position is suitable for *tui na* for the head and face, neck, shoulders, chest, back, and lumbar area.

Lying on one side: The patient should lie down on their side and keep their lower leg straight. The upper leg should be flexed. Similarly, the lower arm should be flexed at 90° at the shoulder and elbow. The upper arm is naturally straight and placed at the side of the body or propped on the bed in front of the patient. This position is suitable for *tui na* for the head, neck, shoulders, upper limbs, chest, ribs, back, waist, hips and lower limbs.

Supine: Remove the pillow or use a low pillow. The patient should lie down face up and place the upper limbs naturally at the side of the body. The lower limbs should be naturally straightened too. The position of the limbs can be adjusted at any time during the massage. This position is suitable for *tui na* for the head, face, neck, chest, abdomen, and lower limbs.

Prone: Remove the pillow and have the patient lie prone with their head tilted to the side. Keep both the lower limbs naturally straight and place the upper limbs on the side of the body, or with the elbows bent and tucked below the face. The position of the limbs can be adjusted at any time during the massage. This position is suitable for *tui na* for the head, neck, back, waist, hips, and lower limbs.

Surface Media for *Tui Na*

Before commencing the *tui na* massage, it is sometimes necessary to apply lubricant, cream, or powder on the treatment site. This is to ensure that the treatment site will not be damaged during the *tui na* massage. These substances may also have medicinal effects that can penetrate the skin. Different ailments will require specific media. For example, cold syndrome ailments will require a heating medium such as spring onion and ginger water to dispel the cold. Heat syndrome will require a cooling medium such as cold water or alcohol. Ailments related to deficiency syndrome require a nourishing medium such as medicinal wine, while ailments related to excess syndrome require a medium that aids in clearing and purging, such as egg white or safflower oil. A neutral medium such as talcum powder can be used for other general ailments.

Tui Na with Hot Compress

Hot compress can either be dry or wet. Dry hot compress is performed by applying a bag to the treatment area. The bag is filled with salt, sand, earth, and herbs that have been heated up through frying. For wet hot compress, Chinese herbs which can eliminate wind and disperse cold, and can warm and activate meridians are placed in a bag. This bag is tied up and boiled in a pot of water. Once the herbal water is boiled, a towel will be soaked and wrung out, folded into a square, and compressed on the treatment site. When the towel is no longer as warm, it will be exchanged for another towel. Wet hot compress is often used after the to-and-fro rubbing method, where the pores around the area are opened after the massage. The hot towel is then compressed onto the treatment site, and light patting is applied to increase the heat transmission. After the hot compress, safflower oil is applied to enhance the effect. Wet hot compress is commonly used in *tui na* massage, generally after the massage session. This helps to improve the therapeutic effect of the massage, and also relieves the adverse reactions caused by excessive stimulation of the body.

Strength and Duration of *Tui Na* Massage

The strength to be exerted for a *tui na* massage is dependent on the patient, the location of the treatment site, the method used, the medical condition, and the physique of the patient. The basic principle for strength exertion is to guarantee a therapeutic effect while avoiding adverse reactions.

The duration of the *tui na* massage session is also dependent on the medical condition. Ailments associated with internal medicine, gynecology, and chronic stress will require a longer treatment time—usually half an hour or longer. The treatment time for acute soft tissues injuries is usually shorter—usually 10 to 15 minutes, or even shorter. If the treatment goes on for too long, it may aggravate the symptoms.

Tips for *Tui Na* Massage

These tips will help you understand the issues to watch out for during a *tui na* massage session, to yield better results.

• Relax the body and mind. The mind should be concentrated during massage, but should be calm. The body should not be tense, and one must relax physically and mentally.

• Know the acupoints well, especially the most commonly used ones. This will be helpful for the location of acupoints and correct *tui na* methods.

• Use appropriate force, and know how much to exert. Too little force will not have the proper stimulating effect, while too much force can cause fatigue and injuries to the skin surface.

• Perform the massage step by step. The number of repetitions, the force exerted, and the number of acupoints to work on should increase progressively.

• Perseverance. Regardless of what the *tui na* massage is used for, be it healthcare or treatment of chronic diseases, remember that the effects will not be visible in the short term. One must persevere to see the gradual results. Have confidence, patience, and persistence.

4. Things to Note for *Tui Na*

Tui na massage is a common traditional Chinese medicinal treatment that can be performed without tools. It looks like a safe procedure, but as a healthcare treatment it also has indications, contraindications, and precautions. It is important to understand these in order to execute *tui na* appropriately and successfully.

Indications for *Tui Na*

Tui na is a form of physical therapy and an external treatment method in traditional Chinese medicine. It has a positive therapeutic effect on many diseases such as orthopedics, internal medicine, gynecology, pediatrics, and ophthalmology and otorhinolaryngology, and can serve as a form of health care and illness prevention. Conditions that can be prevented through *tui na* are as follows:

Internal illnesses: Stomachache, diarrhea, constipation, headaches, palpitations, hemiplegia, cold, coughing, asthma, and insomnia.

Gynecological disorders: Irregular menstruation, menstrual pain, amenorrhea, and morbid leucorrhea.

Male diseases: Nocturnal emission and impotence.

Orthopedic disorders: Neck pain, stiff neck, tendon injuries of the limb joints, lumbago, and rheumatic arthritis.

Pediatric diseases: Infant diarrhea, vomiting, abdominal pain, constipation, fever, cough, enuresis, fright, and night crying.

Ophthalmology and otorhinolaryngology diseases: Myopia, toothache, sinusitis, and sore throat.

To conclude, the application of *tui na* is very wide. It can be used for the prevention and treatment of chronic illnesses, and is also used to prevent and treat some acute diseases. Its application is not limited to a certain stage of illness; it can also be used to treat these diseases in general.

Contraindications to *Tui Na*

To avoid adverse effects, *tui na* should not be performed in the following cases:

Patients suffering from acute and chronic infectious diseases such as measles, tuberculosis, and polio.

Patients suffering from orthopedic diseases such as fractures, joint dislocation, bone and joint tuberculosis, bone tumors, and osteomyelitis.

Patients with severe heart disease, liver disease, and kidney disease.

Patients suffering from malignant tumors, severe anemia, or long-standing illnesses and extreme weakness.

Patients who suffer from thrombocytopenic purpura, allergic purpura, or hemophilia.

Patients with skin problems, large surface areas of skin lesions, or ulcerative dermatitis.

Menstruating and pregnant women. *Tui na* massage should not be used on some areas.

Tui na massage should not be performed right after a shower, strenuous exercise, or consuming alcohol. It is not suitable for patients who have hyperpyrexia or over fatigue, or who are either starving or over-sated.

Precautions for *Tui Na*

Patients who are in the early stage of a severe acute injury, or are experiencing severe swelling should only have *tui na* on local areas 24 to 72 hours after sustaining the injury. This is to prevent aggravation and local internal bleeding.

For acute injuries, it is not advisable to apply hot compress to the local area during the *tui na* treatment to avoid interstitial oedema, especially for the first treatment.

Patients who receive their first *tui na* treatment may suffer from local aggravation of symptoms 1 to 2 days after. This is only temporary, and will go away on its own after 2 to 3 days, so there is no need to worry.

In addition to the above precautions, you should also be mindful of the duration of the *tui na* massage. Ideally, each session should be 20 minutes long. It is also advisable to perform *tui na* massage once in the morning and once at night, e.g., after waking in the morning and before turning in at night. Try to have direct contact with the skin during the massage. If you sweat after the massage, you should pay attention to avoid wind so as not to catch a cold.

Handling Abnormalities during *Tui Na*

Fainting: If the patient faints during treatment, stop immediately. Put the patient in a ventilated place and give them some plain or sugared water.

Bruises: Treatment is not necessary for minor bruises. However, if the local bruising is severe, cold compress or elastic bandages can be applied with pressure first. After the hemorrhage stops, gentle *tui na* massage can be applied on the local area, together with wet hot compress to reduce swelling and relieve pain.

Abrasion: When rubbing and kneading, the patient's skin may be damaged. In this situation, stop immediately, and disinfect the affected area to prevent infection.

Pain: Pain arising from *tui na* massage does not usually require any special treatment, and will fade on its own within 1 to 2 days. If the pain is more intense, apply Fotalin (diclofenac diethylamine emulsion) ointment. In the early stage, cold compress can be applied to the local area. Subsequently, light *tui na* methods such as kneading, circular rubbing and pressing and wet hot compress can be used.

Fatigue: A small group of people will feel tired and dull after *tui na* massage. Most people with these symptoms are deficient in *qi* and blood, and may have symptoms such as poor gastrointestinal absorption and weak constitution. Drinking an infusion of ginger, red dates, and longan can help regulate their *qi* and blood, and can reduce discomfort during the *tui na* treatment.

5. Locating Commonly Used Acupoints

Acupoints are special parts of the body where the surface, deep tissues, and organs are closely connected. They are distributed in a point-like manner across the surface of the body. They are not isolated points, but are located where nerve endings are dense or where nerve fibers pass. According to traditional Chinese medicine, they reflect the infusion of *qi* and blood from the internal meridians. They can be regarded as the reaction points for disease, the stimulation points for treatment, and the sensitive points for beauty. Therefore, they are crucial in acupuncture and massage. There are four main methods used for locating acupoints: anatomical landmarks, proportional bone measurement, finger-cun measurement, and simplified measurement.

Anatomical Landmarks

This method is based on various surface markers, either fixed or active.

Fixed markers: The protrusions and depressions formed by the bones and muscles of the various body parts, as well as the outline of the sensory organs, hairline, nails, nipples, and armpits can be taken as acupoint marks. For example, the Yintang acupoint is located between the eyebrows. The Danzhong acupoint is located in between the nipples, and the Yanglingquan acupoint is located at the depression point at the head of the fibula (at the lateral part of the calf).

Active markers: Active markers refer to the gaps, depressions, wrinkles, and tips of the joints, muscles, tendons and skin during movement and activity. For example, the Quchi acupoint is located at the depression of the cubital crease when the elbow is flexed, while the Tinggong acupoint is found in the depression between the antilobium and temporomandibular joint when the mouth is open.

Proportional Bone Measurement

This method uses bone joints as the main mark to determine the length of the bones and according to its proportional conversion as the standard for determining the point. Based on this method, proportional conversion is the same regardless of sex, age, height, or physique, resolving the issue of different people having different acupoint locations.

Body Part	Starting and Ending Points	Bone Length (cun)	Direction of Measure
Head and face	Middle of anterior hairline to middle of posterior hairline	12	Vertical
	Between the eyebrows (Yintang acupoint) to middle of the front hairline	3	Vertical
	Between the two frontal hairline (Touwei acupoints)	9	Horizontal
	Between the two mastoids behind the ears (Wan'gu acupoints)	9	Horizontal

Body Part	Starting and Ending Points	Bone Length (cun)	Direction of Measure
Thorax, abdomen, and hypo-chondrium	Suprasternal fossa (Tiantu acupoint) to midpoint of xiphisternal synchondrosis	9	Vertical
	Midpoint of xiphisternal synchondrosis to belly button (Shenque acupoint)	8	Vertical
	Belly button (Shenque acupoint) to upper margin of pubic symphysis (Qugu acupoint)	5	Vertical
	Between the two nipples	8	Horizontal
	Between the medial edge of both coracoid process of scapula	12	Horizontal
Lumbar back	Medial border of scapula to posterior median line	3	Horizontal
Upper limbs	Anterior and posterior axillary fold to cubital crease (parallel to olecranon)	9	Vertical
	Cubital crease (parallel to olecranon) to anterior (dorsal) carpal distal crease	12	Vertical
Lower limbs	Upper margin of pubic symphysis (Qugu acupoint) to base of patella	18	Vertical
	Base of patella to apex of patella	2	Vertical
	Apex of patella (mid-knee) to prominence of medial malleolus	15	Vertical
	Below the condylus medialis tibiae (Yinlingquan acupoint) to prominence of medial malleolus	13	Vertical
	Greater trochanter of femur to popliteal transverse line (parallel to apex of patella)	19	Vertical
	Gluteal sulcus to popliteal transverse line	14	Vertical
	Popliteal transverse line (parallel to apex of patella) to prominence of lateral malleolus	16	Vertical
	Prominence of medial malleolus to sole	3	Vertical

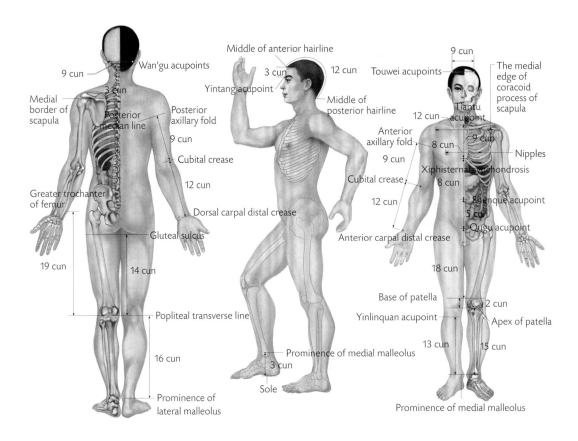

Labels on left figure (posterior view):
- 9 cun
- Wan'gu acupoints
- 3 cun
- Medial border of scapula
- Posterior median line
- Posterior axillary fold
- 9 cun
- Cubital crease
- 12 cun
- Dorsal carpal distal crease
- Greater trochanter of femur
- Gluteal sulcus
- 19 cun
- 14 cun
- Popliteal transverse line
- 16 cun
- Prominence of lateral malleolus

Labels on middle figure (lateral view):
- Middle of anterior hairline
- 3 cun
- 12 cun
- Yintang acupoint
- Middle of posterior hairline
- 9 cun
- Cubital crease
- 12 cun
- Anterior carpal distal crease
- Prominence of medial malleolus
- 3 cun
- Sole

Labels on right figure (anterior view):
- 9 cun
- Touwei acupoints
- The medial edge of coracoid process of scapula
- Tiantu acupoint
- 12 cun
- 8 cun
- 9 cun
- Anterior axillary fold
- Nipples
- 9 cun
- Xiphisternal synchondrosis
- Cubital crease
- 8 cun
- 12 cun
- Shenque acupoint
- 5 cun
- Qugu acupoint
- 18 cun
- Base of patella
- 2 cun
- Yinlinquan acupoint
- Apex of patella
- 13 cun
- 15 cun
- Prominence of medial malleolus

Finger-Cun Measurement

Acupoints can be located using the length and width of a person's finger.

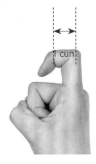

1 cun

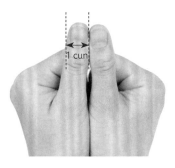

1 cun

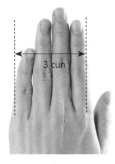

3 cun

Use middle finger length: The distance between the two inner ends of two cross striation when the middle finger is placed on the body for location of acupoint is 1 cun. This placement method can be used on the lower back and the four limbs.

Use thumb length: The lateral width of the interphalangeal joint of the thumb is taken to be 1 cun. This placement method is commonly used on the four limbs.

Use four fingers closed together: With the index finger, middle finger, ring finger, and small finger of the patient stretched straight and closed, measure at the level of the large knuckle (the second joint) of the middle finger. The width of the four fingers is 3 cun.

Simplified Measurement

This is a commonly used method to locate acupoints easily. Although it is not applicable to all acupoints, it is easy to execute and remember.

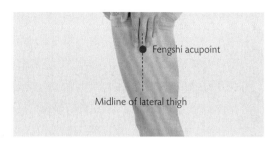

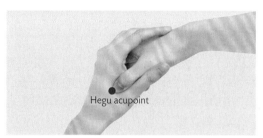

Fengshi acupoint: Stand up straight and let the hands hang down naturally to each side. Keep the fingers closed. The acupoint is located at the tip of the middle finger.

Hegu acupoint: Align the transverse line of the thumb of one hand with the web between the thumb and index finger of the other hand. The acupoint is located at the tip of the thumb.

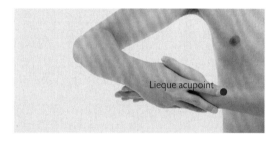

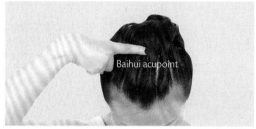

Lieque acupoint: Intersect the web between the thumb and index finger of both hands. Press the styloid process of radius of one hand with the index finger. The acupoint is located at the tip of the index finger.

Baihui acupoint: The point where the two ear tips and the middle of the head intersect has a slight depression when pressed. This acupoint is located at the depression.

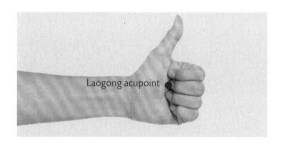

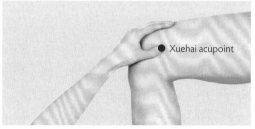

Laogong acupoint: Clench your fist and press the palm with the middle finger. The acupoint point is located at the first cross striation of the palm where the tip of the middle finger is pressing on.

Xuehai acupoint: Bend your knee 90° and place your palm on it. Form a 45° angle with the thumb and the other fingers. The acupoint is located at the tip of the thumb.

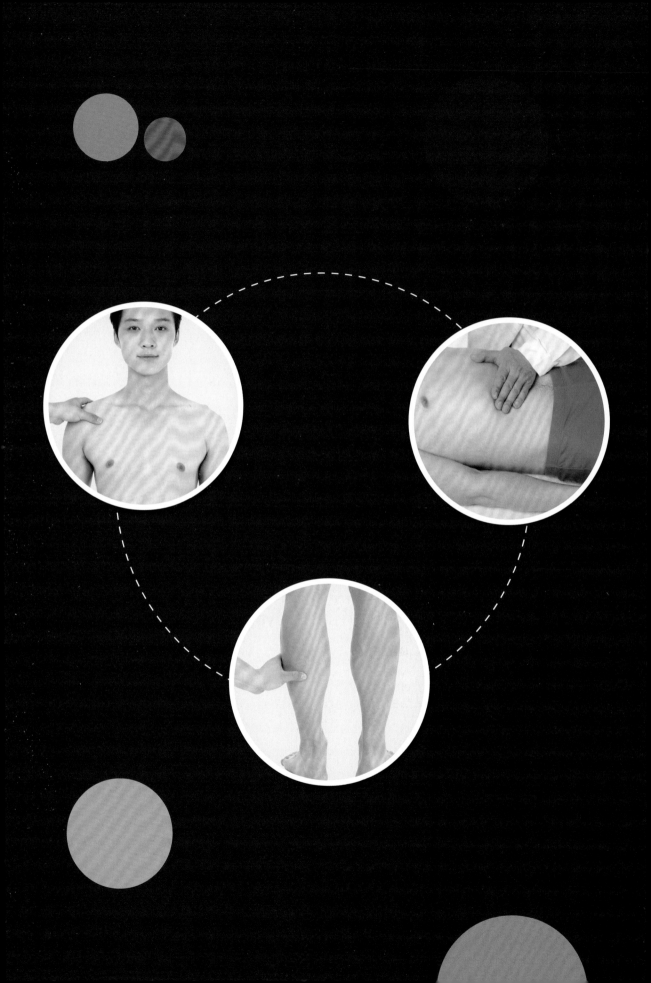

CHAPTER TWO
Alleviating Body Aches and Pains through *Tui Na*

Fatigue, sports injuries, bone aging, and lowered immunity are some causes of poor blood circulation, which in turn causes joint pain. It is common for office workers, athletes, the middle aged, and the elderly to suffer pain in areas such as the neck, shoulders, waist, and legs. *Tui na* can help to dredge meridians, accelerate blood circulation, regulate the recovery of injured soft tissue, and release adhesion. It is an effective way to relieve muscle and joint pain caused by the various ailments. It can also help regulate the body, improve physical fitness, alleviate soreness and pain, and allows you to enjoy a more relaxed body.

Note: Some photographs in the book do not have acupoints marked out due to the angle at which the photographs were taken. Please refer to the appendix for the list of commonly used acupoints in *tui na*. You may wish to follow through the step-by-step instructions or use some of them based on your body condition. Massage both acupoints if they are symmetrically distributed on the body.

1. Stiff Neck

Stiff neck is characterized by sudden neck pain and limited neck mobility. Its occurrence is often related to factors such as bad sleeping posture, uncomfortable pillow height, excessive pressure on the neck, and cold pathogen.

Tui na duration: 2 to 3 minutes for each acupoint.

Principles of treatment: To relax the tendons, dredge the collaterals, and regulate the recovery of injured soft tissue.

Points to note: Incorporate neck mobility exercises to daily life upon recovery, and pay attention to the protection of the neck, so as to minimize the chances of reoccurrence.

Steps

❶ Pinching-grasping and pressing-kneading methods: Have the patient seated in an upright position. Apply the five-finger pinching-grasping method on the patient's neck for 30 to 50 times. Thereafter, press and knead the patient's Fengchi and Fengfu acupoints for 2 to 3 minutes each, using the pulp of either the index finger or the thumb.

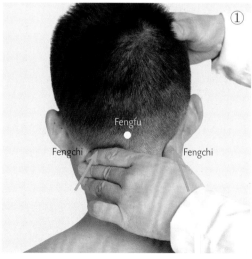

❷ Rolling and kneading methods: Have the patient seated in an upright position. First apply the rolling and kneading methods on the patient's neck and shoulder for about 2 to 3 minutes. Next, perform light stretching on the neck to relieve muscle tension. (Apply light force during *tui na*, and keep the neck relaxed).

❸ Plucking method: Use the thumb to flick Jianzhongshu acupoint for a minute, and pluck the area that experiences muscle spasm. It is appropriate for the patient to have a feeling of soreness and swelling.

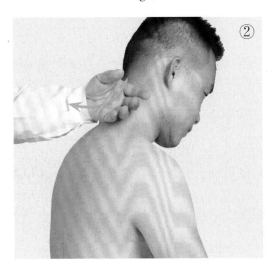

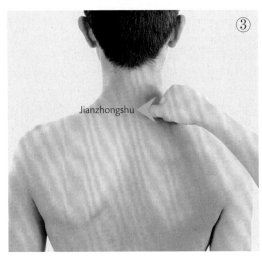

Jianzhongshu

❹ Stretching method: Have the patient seated upright. Stand behind the patient and hold the back of the patient's head. Hold the patient's jaw with the upper limb of the other hand with the elbow bend. Support the side of the patient's head with the palm. Pull the head upwards with both hands simultaneously to stretch the cervical vertebrae. This method should be applied gently.

❺ Pulling method: Have the patient seated in an upright position with their neck relaxed. Place one hand on the back of the patient's head and the other on the chin. Rotate the patient's head slightly from side to side. When the neck is fully relaxed, use obliquely pulling method to do a quick pull to the affected area. A popping sound will be heard.

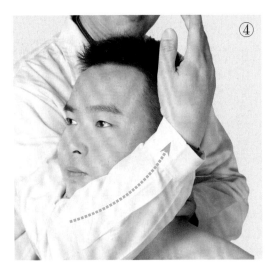

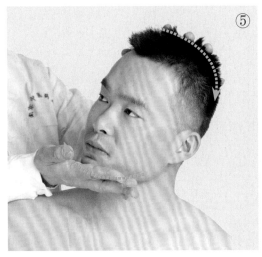

2. Cervical Spondylosis

Cervical spondylosis is a common ailment among middle-aged and elderly people. The condition is caused when cervical vertebral hyperplasia stimulates or compresses the cervical nerve root, cervical spinal cord, vertebral artery, or sympathetic nerve. For mild cases, the head, neck, shoulders and arms are numb and painful. In severe cases, the limbs are sore and weak, and the patient will suffer from incontinence and paralysis.

Tui na duration: 2 to 3 minutes for each acupoint.

Principles of treatment: To relax the tendons, promote blood circulation, and to regulate the recovery of injured soft tissue.

Points to note: Patients with vertebral artery cervical spondylosis should not perform backward head-turning exercises to avoid aggravating the symptoms of vertigo.

Steps

❶ Rolling method: Have the patient seated upright. Use the rolling method or finger-pushing method from behind. Apply slight force to the patient's shoulders for 2 to 3 minutes.

❷ Pressing-kneading and pinching-grasping methods: Press-knead Fengfu, Fengchi and Tianzong acupoints with the thumb or index finger in a clockwise or counter clockwise direction for 2 to 3 minutes each. Thereafter, pinch-grasp the Fengchi acupoint with the thumb and index finger for about 2 minutes.

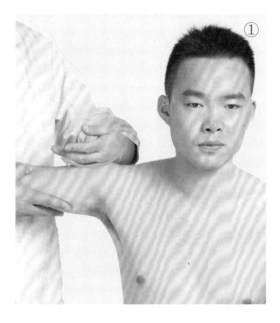
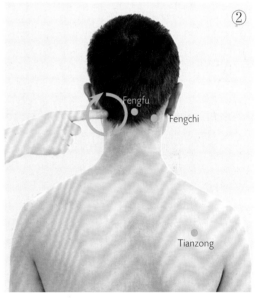

❸ Pressing-kneading method: Press-knead the Shousanli acupoint using the thumb or index finger in a clockwise direction for 2 to 3 minutes. This method should ideally cause slight soreness.

❹ Rotating method: Have the patient seated in an upright position with the neck relaxed. Either stand behind or on the side of the patient. Hold the patient's head from the back with one hand and hold the chin with the other. Rotate the head slowly left and right with force.

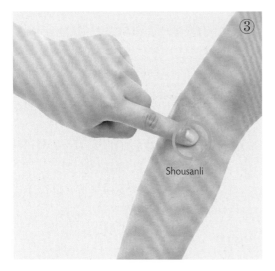

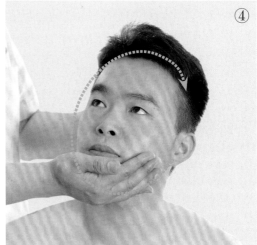

Shousanli

5 Stretching method: Have the patient seated upright. Stand behind the patient and hold the back of their head. Support the head with the other hand by supporting the lower jaw with the elbow and the palm of the hand on the posterior occipital region. Exert a slow pulling force upwards while bending the elbow to stretch the patient's cervical spine.

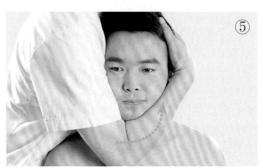

3. Frozen Shoulder

Frozen shoulder is an inflammatory reaction of the soft tissues around the shoulder joint, including muscles, tendons, bursa, and joint capsule, caused by degenerative changes in the joint and its surrounding soft tissues. Frozen shoulder is a common and frequent ailment among the middle-aged and elderly. Its main symptom is a radiating pain in the shoulder.

Tui na **duration:** 2 to 3 minutes for each acupoint.

Principles of treatment: To relax the tendons, and dredge the collaterals.

Points to note: Keep the shoulder warm. Avoid catching cold and overexertion.

Steps

1 Rolling and kneading methods: Have the patient seated upright. Those who are frail or are suffering from other ailments can lie on their back. Apply the rolling and kneading methods on the affected shoulder or upper limb for treatment, and incorporate abduction activities on the affected limb. Note: Apply *tui na* first before performing the abduction exercises.

2 Pressing-kneading and grasping methods: Press-knead the Tianzong, Bingfeng and Jianyu acupoints on both sides 5 to 10 times each using the thumb or index finger. Next, apply the grasping method on the Jianjing acupoint for 2 to 3 minutes. This step should ideally produce a sore and numb feeling on the shoulder.

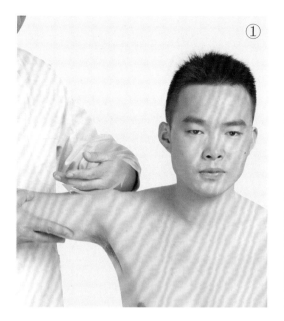
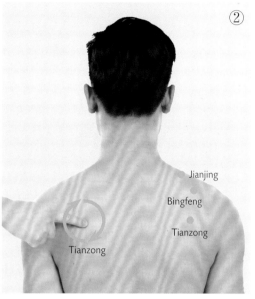

Jianjing

Bingfeng

Tianzong

Tianzong

❸ Single finger meditation pushing and plucking methods: Apply the single finger meditation pushing method on the bicep tendon, and incorporate some light abduction activities. Next, apply the plucking method on the inter-nodal groove and the bicep tendon. Note that the action should be gentle.

❹ Rotating and stretching methods: Apply the rotating method on the shoulder for about one minute. Next, stretch the shoulder joint.

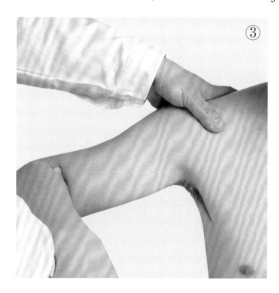
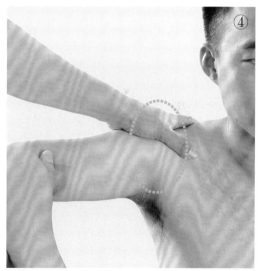

❺ To-and-fro rubbing method: Have the patient seated in an upright position with the shoulder relaxed. Stand on the right of the patient. Apply the to-and-fro rubbing method to the shoulder with thenar to generate heat for penetration.

❻ Palm twisting and pulling-shaking methods: Apply the palm twisting method with both palms, and rub the patient's upper limbs until the skin is flushed. Next, pull-shake the limb for about one minute.

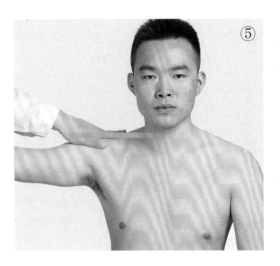

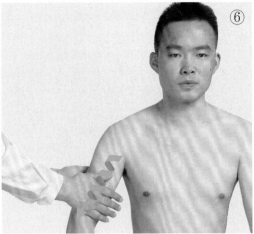

4. Shoulder Joint Sprain

....

When the soft tissues of the human shoulder are injured by a blow or collision, or by pulling or twisting, it is called a shoulder sprain. This injury can occur at any age. It is characterized by a closed injury, and is located mostly on the upper or lateral side of the shoulder.

Tui na **duration:** 2 to 3 minutes for each acupoint.

Principles of treatment: To promote blood circulation to remove meridian obstruction, and to regulate the recovery of injured soft tissue.

Points to note: Avoid strenuous abduction and external rotation of the shoulder during activities.

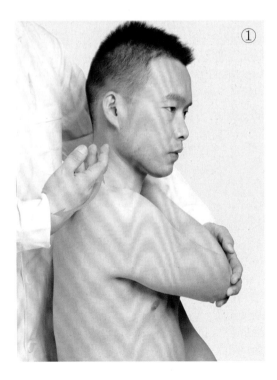

Steps

❶ Rolling method: Have the patient seated in an upright position, with shoulders slightly drooped and curled in. Keeping the shoulder relaxed, apply the rolling method on the supraspinatus muscle for two minutes.

❷ Finger pressing, and pinching-grasping methods: Have the patient seated in an upright position. Apply either the finger pressing or pressing-kneading method on the deltoid area of the affected shoulder 50 times. Next, apply the pinching-grasping method on the deltoid muscle for 2 to 3 minutes using the thumb and index finger.

❸ Plucking and pinching-grasping methods: Apply the plucking method on the stiff shoulder area 3 to 5 times. Alternatively use the pinching-grasping method to relieve the shoulder spasm, eliminate stasis, and alleviate pain.

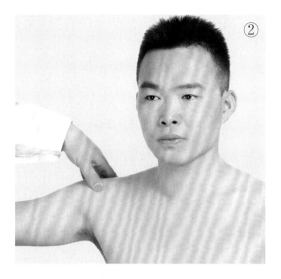

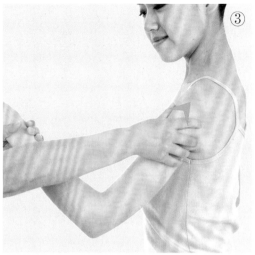

❹ Rotating method: Have the patient seated upright. Hold the patient's shoulder with one hand and the wrist with the other. Flex the arm to rotate the shoulder. The amplitude of rotation can be from small to large. Repeat this method 5 to 7 times.

❺ Pulling-shaking and grasping-kneading methods: Have the patient seated in an upright position. Apply the pulling-shaking method to the patient's shoulder while performing some gentle grasping-kneading movements. Note that the patient should not hold their breath during this *tui na* massage.

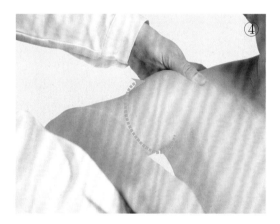

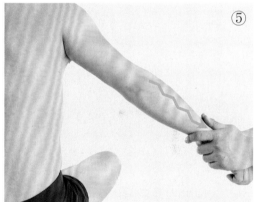

5. Rheumatic Lower Back Pain

Rheumatic lower back pain is caused by the pathogenic wind, cold, and damp on the lower back region, resulting in numbing and congested blood vessels and poor circulation, thus causing symptoms such as soreness, pain, and numbness in the lower back region. This ailment is associated with fatigue, getting cold, and humidity.

Tui na duration: 2 to 3 minutes for each acupoint.

Principles of treatment: To relax the tendons and promote blood circulation.

Points to note: Do not stand or sit for long periods of time; maintain moderate activity.

Steps

❶ Rolling method: Have the patient lying in a prone position. Stand on one side and apply the rolling method up and down along the Taiyang Bladder Meridian of Foot on both sides of the patient's waist 5 to 6 times. This method is a more stimulatory one. The force should be great so that the patient can feel the stimulation.

❷ Finger pressing method: Use the pulp of index finger to finger press on the patient's Mingmen, Qihaishu, and Guanyuanshu acupoints. Alternatively, press Jiaji acupoints on both sides of the spine using the palms. Each acupoint should be pressed for about two minutes. This method can also be operated with the thumb pulp.

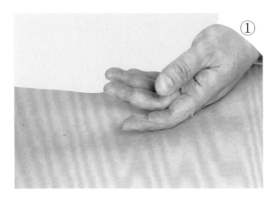
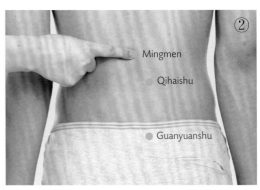

Mingmen

Qihaishu

Guanyuanshu

❸ Pressing method: Have the patient lying in a prone position. Press on the Dachangshu and the Baliao acupoints using both thumbs, ideally to generate soreness. The pressure used for this method can be slightly greater.

❹ Pushing and to-and-fro rubbing methods: Rub the Taiyang Bladder Meridian of Foot on both sides of the back directly with hypothenar or the entire palm, followed by pushing and rubbing the lumbosacral area until the heat has penetrated the skin.

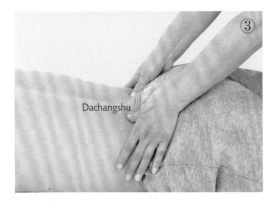
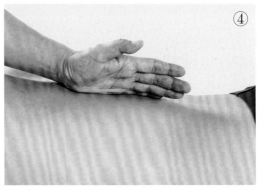

Dachangshu

❺ Patting method: Have the patient lying in a prone position. Use the palm to pat the sacrospinalis on both sides of the lower back to the extent that the skin is slightly flushed. For patients who experience soreness and pain, hot compress can be applied to the affected area.

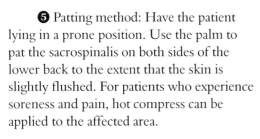
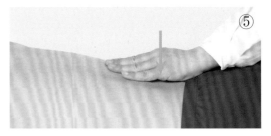

6. Lumbar Muscle Strain

Lumbar muscle strain is a chronic inflammation of the lumbar muscles and their attachment points of the fascia or periosteum. It is one of the common causes of lumbar pain. The main symptoms are swelling and soreness in the lumbar or lumbosacral region, with recurring episodes. The pain can change with the climate or varying degrees of exertion. For example, pain can be intensified from exerting muscles in the day, but it can be alleviated after rest.

Tui na **duration:** 3 to 5 minutes for each body part.

Principles of treatment: To relax the tendons, dredge the collaterals, and to promote blood circulation and remove blood stasis.

Points to note: Train to strengthen back muscles and participate in outdoor activities moderately.

Steps

❶ Rolling and kneading methods: Have the patient lying in a prone position. Stand on one side and apply the heavy rolling and kneading methods up and down the lumbosacral area 5 to 6 times. The force exerted should increase from light to heavy.

❷ Finger pressing method: Have the patient lying in a prone position. Press on the Shenshu and Dachangshu acupoints for one minute each, followed by stretching of the waist. This method has the effect of dispersing stasis and promoting blood circulation to alleviate pain.

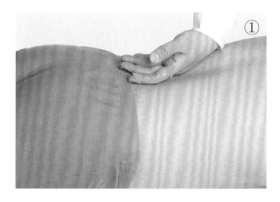

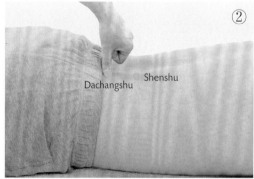

❸ Pulling method: Have the patient lying on the side. Stand facing the patient and apply waist side pulling method once on the lumbar region for each side. This method should be applied in a steady, accurate, and light manner. Do not overexert with this method.

❹ Rotating method: Have the patient lying in a supine position with their knees and hips tucked in. Hold their knees and perform the lumbosacral rotation clockwise and anti-clockwise 8 to 10 times each. The speed of the rotation should be slow.

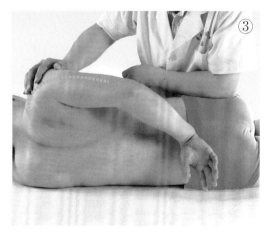

❺ To-and-fro rubbing method: Rub the Taiyang Bladder Meridian of Foot on both sides of the patient's lower back directly with hypothenar, and then rub the lumbosacral region transversely to let the heat penetrate.

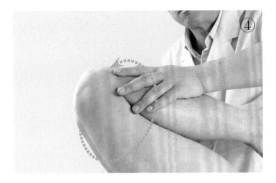
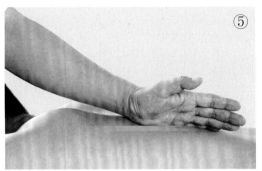

7. Acute Lumbar Sprain

Acute lumbar sprain is an acute laceration of the lumbar muscles, fascia, ligaments, and other soft tissues caused by sudden overstretching due to external forces. It often occurs when lifting heavy objects and during strong contractions of the lumbar muscles. An acute lumbar sprain can tear the attachment points of the lumbosacral muscles, periosteum, fascia, ligaments, and other tissues.

Tui na **duration:** Approximately one minute for each acupoint.

Principles of treatment: To relax the tendons and promote blood circulation, and to regulate the recovery of injured soft tissue.

Points to note: Keep the affected area warm, and focus on lumbar strengthening exercises after the pain is gone.

Steps
❶ Rolling method: Have the patient lying in a prone position with the limbs relaxed. Stand on the affected side and apply the rolling or pressing-kneading method on the sacrospinal muscles on both sides of the lumbar vertebrae 3 to 5 times each. This method can relieve the discomfort of the lumbar region.

❷ Finger pressing method: Use both thumbs to press on the Yaoyangguan, Shenshu, Qihaishu, and Dachangshu acupoints for one minute each. The force exerted should go from light to heavy, and this method should produce soreness.

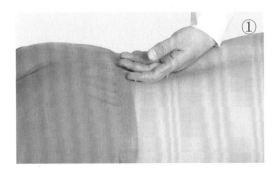
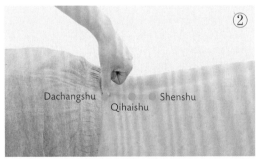

❸ Grasping and kneading methods: Use the thumb and index finger to hold and knead the Weizhong acupoint (middle point of the popliteal fossa) with relative force to produce soreness.

❹ Plucking method: Have the patient lying in a prone position. Apply the plucking method on the areas with pain and spasms. This method should be executed in a gentle manner, 3 to 5 times in each area.

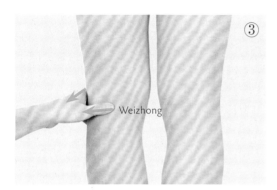
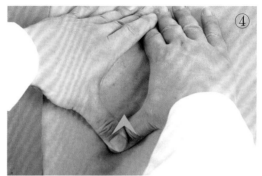

❺ Pulling and rotating methods: Press the lumbosacral area with one palm and hold the lower 1/3 of the thigh on one side of the patient with the other hand. Apply the pulling method and pull upwards as much as possible 5 to 8 times. Then shake and rotate the patient's lumbosacral region and hip, a few times each.

❻ To-and-fro rubbing method: Have the patient lying in a prone position. Apply the to-and-fro rubbing method with hypothenar on the injured side, along the direction of sacrospinalis fibers until the heat generated penetrates the skin.

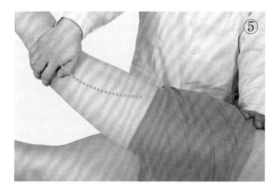
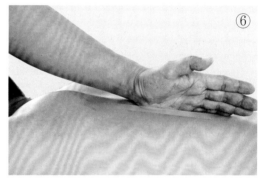

8. Lumbar Disc Herniation

Lumbar intervertebral disc herniation is one of the common ailments, mainly because of the varying degrees of degenerative changes in the lumbar intervertebral disc. Due to external pressure, the fibrous ring of the lumbar intervertebral disc ruptures and the nucleus pulposus tissue protrudes (or dislocates) from the rupture in the posterior or vertebral canal, resulting in stimulation or compression of the adjacent spinal nerve roots. This can cause a series of clinical symptoms such as lumbar pain, numbness, and pain in one or both lower limbs.

Tui na duration: Approximately 2 to 3 minutes for each area.

Principles of treatment: To relax the tendons, dredge the collaterals, and to promote blood circulation and remove blood stasis.

Points to note: Maintain a good sitting posture. Avoid sleeping on beds that are too soft. People who are desk bound for a long period of time should pay attention to the height of the table and chair, and maintain a correct sitting posture.

Steps

❶ Rolling method: Have the patient lying in a prone position. Stand on one side and apply the gentle rolling method on the waist, hips, and lower limbs. Repeat 3 to 5 times to relax the muscles.

❷ Pressing-kneading method: Have the patient lying in a prone position. Apply the pressing-kneading method on the Yaoyangguan, Shenshu, Dachangshu, and Huantiao acupoints for 2 to 3 minutes each. This method should produce soreness.

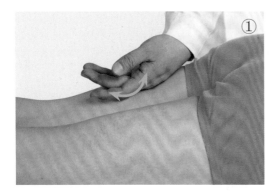
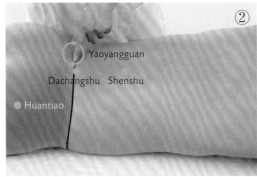

❸ Vibrating method: Have the patient lying in a prone position. Stack your left palm on your right palm, and apply a downward rhythmic pressure on the waist, so that it vibrates. The force and the pressure applied should gradually increase from light to heavy. Relax, and repeat this method for 1 to 2 minutes.

❹ Pulling method: Have the patient side lying with the affected area on top. Stand in front of the patient. Press one hand on the shoulder and pull forward and downwards. Press the other hand or elbow on top of the hip and press backward and downwards. Both hands should exert force at the same time, and it is common to hear a clicking sound coming from the waist.

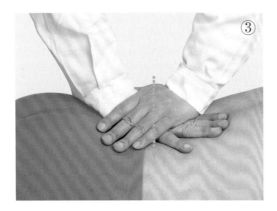
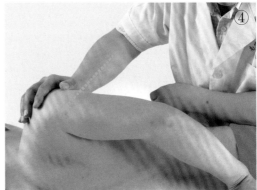

❺ Pulling method: Have the patient side lying. Stand on one side of the patient. Hold on to their top knee and lift it upwards. Keep the other hand firmly pressed on the affected lumbar area. When the waist is stretched to its maximum, pull both hands simultaneously in the opposite direction.

❻ To-and-fro rubbing: Have the patient lying in a prone position. Use the pressure pain point as the center of reference, and rub the lumbosacral area with hypothenar until the heat generated penetrates the skin.

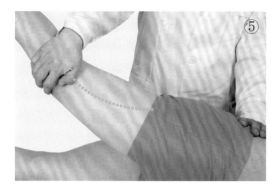
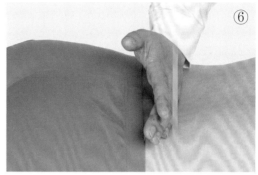

9. Sciatica

Sciatica is characterized by pain in the main trunk and distribution area of the sciatic nerve. The vast majority of cases of sciatica are secondary to irritation, compression, and damage to the sciatic nerve by lesions of the local and surrounding structures.

Tui na duration: Approximately 2 to 3 minutes for each affected area.

Principles of treatment: To relax the tendons and promote blood circulation.

Points to note: Patients suffering from sciatica are advised to sleep on hard beds.

Steps

❶ Pressing-kneading method: Use the pulp of index finger or thumb to press the Zhibian and Huantiao acupoints. Press firmly in a clockwise direction for 2 to 3 minutes. Localized soreness and swelling may be felt or a trickling numbness radiating to the lower extremities.

❷ Pressing-kneading method: Use the pulp of index finger or thumb to press the Juliao acupoint forcefully. Gradually increase the force applied and the depth of depression for 2 to 3 minutes.

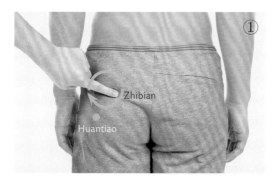
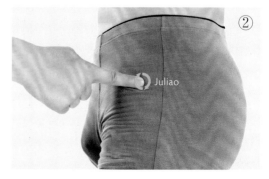

❸ Pressing-kneading method: Use thumb pulp to press the Chengfu acupoint for about two minutes. This method should produce soreness.

❹ Pressing-kneading method: Use thumb pulp to press the Chengshan acupoint for about one minute. This method should produce soreness.

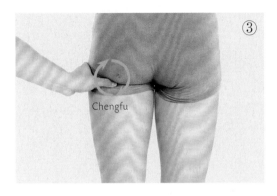

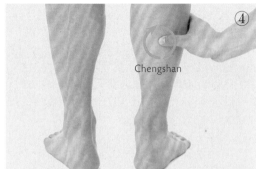

❺ Striking method: Strike the Yaoshu acupoint with a fist about ten times. The force applied can be slightly stronger.

❻ Pressing method: Press the Yinmen, Yaoshu, and Dachangshu acupoints about 20 times with the pulp of index finger. This method should produce soreness.

❼ Pushing method: Use the thumb pulp to push from between the first and second toe up towards the Taichong acupoint about 20 times. The force can be slightly heavier.

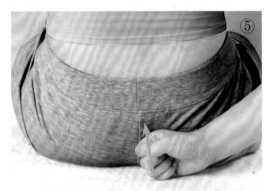

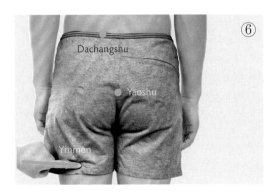

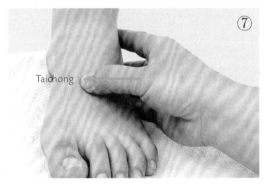

10. Postpartum Lumbago

Postpartum lumbago is a condition in which women experience lumbosacral pain after delivery on either or both sides of the waist, sometimes triggering leg pain. It is aggravated by exertion and can be relieved after a rest.

Tui na **duration:** Approximately two minutes for each affected area.

Principles of treatment: To relax the tendons, dredge the collaterals, and to promote blood circulation and remove blood stasis.

Points to note: Patients should not overexert themselves or do laborious work. Instead, they should take more rest.

Steps

❶ Rolling method: Have the patient lying in a prone position. Apply the rolling method around the treatment site, gradually moving towards the area of pain. Roll in the direction of the sacrospinalis fibers 3 to 4 times, and incorporate lumbar stretching exercises. The amplitude should increase, and the force applied should intensify.

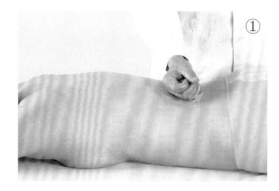

❷ Pressing-kneading method: Have the patient lying in a prone position. Press the Shenshu acupoint and place the other hand on top. Press-knead in a clockwise direction. The force exerted should intensify, and the treatment site should ideally feel sore from this method.

❸ Plucking method: Have the patient lying in a prone position. Apply the plucking method on the top and bottom of the area of pain. The plucking should be light and gentle.

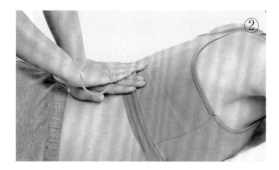

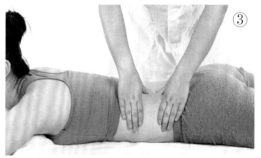

❹ Pulling method: Have the patient side lying. Put one hand on their shoulder and the other arm on their hip, rotating the waist to the maximum. Both hands should then simultaneously pull in the opposite direction. The pulling action must be gentle.

❺ To-and-fro rubbing method: Have the patient lying in a prone position. Rub their lumbosacral region with the palm transversely until the heat generated penetrates the skin.

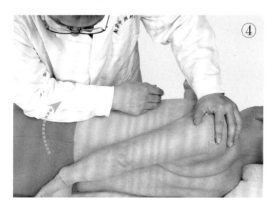

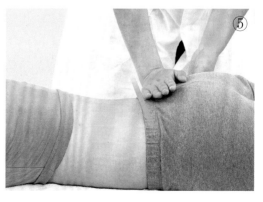

11. Tenosynovitis

The tendon sheath is a synovial sheath that protects the tendon and is wrapped around the tendon in two layers, with synovial fluid between the two layers. When the tendon rubs excessively for a long time, the tendon and the tendon sheath can be damaged by inflammation, causing swelling, called tenosynovitis.

Tui na duration: Approximately two minutes for each affected area.

Principles of treatment: To relax the tendons, dredge the collaterals, and to promote blood circulation and remove blood stasis.

Points to note: During the treatment period, do not overexert the injured hand, and avoid cold stimulation.

Steps

❶ Pressing-kneading method: Have the patient sitting upright with their dorsal carpal facing upwards. Press and knead the radial styloid (the raised bone on the thumb side of the wrist) with the thumb pulp 3 to 5 times. Note that this method should be gentle.

❷ Pushing method: Have the patient sitting upright with their dorsal carpal facing upwards. Hold the injured hand with one hand, and use the thumb of the other hand to push down along the radial styloid 5 to 10 times. The amplitude should gradually increase.

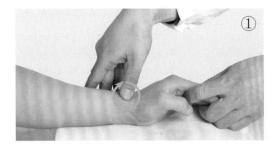 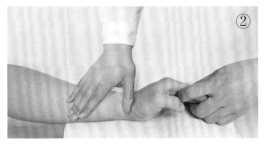

❸ Stretching method: Hold the distal phalanges of the affected finger with the index and middle fingers of one hand, and the proximal end of the metacarpophalangeal joint of the affected limb with the other hand. Apply the stretching method in the opposite direction. Note that the movements should be gentle, and brute force should not be used.

❹ Rotating method: Use the index and middle fingers of one hand to hold the proximal segment of the affected thumb, while the other hand grasps the affected part. Two hands pull against each other while doing adduction, abduction and rotation of the affected wrist. Note that the movements should be gentle.

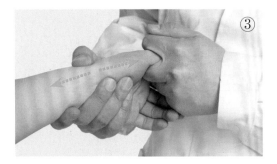 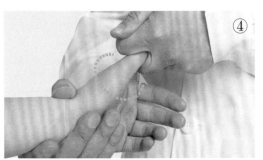

❺ Holding-twisting method: Hold the wrist of the affected limb with one hand, and pinch the metacarpophalangeal joint of the affected limb with the thumb and index finger of the other hand. Twist the affected finger from the inside and outwards. The twisting motion should be fast. Repeat this for approximately two minutes.

❻ To-and-fro rubbing method: Hold the fingers of the affected limb with one hand. Start rubbing to-and-fro with the other hand. The direction of rubbing should be a straight line from the dorsal side of the first metacarpal to the forearm. Repeat this until the heat generated penetrates the skin.

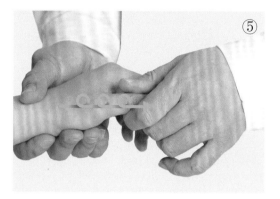
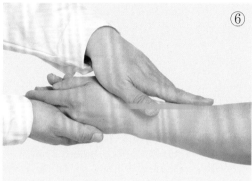

12. Carpal Tunnel Syndrome

With computers getting more common, people often need to use screens, keyboards, and mice for a long period of time in offices and study rooms. This leads to excessive strain on the hands, and over time carpal tunnel syndrome can develop—a condition in which the median nerve in the carpal tunnel of the wrist is compressed and causes numbness and dysfunction of the fingers.

Tui na duration: Approximately two minutes for each affected area.

Principles of treatment: To relax the tendons, dredge the collaterals, and to promote blood circulation and remove blood stasis.

Points to note: Choose a suitable mouse and mouse pad to relieve pressure on the wrist joint when using a computer for a long time. Do not maintain a single posture for too long, and avoid overexertion of the fingers and wrist. Do stretching exercises for the hands and wrists.

Steps

❶ Pressing-kneading method: Use the pulp of thumb or index finger to press-knead the Quze, Neiguan, and Daling acupoints until the patient feels soreness.

❷ Single finger meditation pushing method: Apply this method on the forearm to the hand along the Jueyin Pericardium Meridian of Hand, pushing to-and-fro.

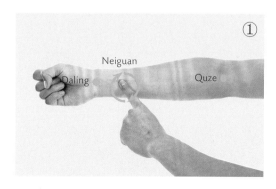

Apply more force on the carpal tunnel and thenar, starting off light and gradually increasing.

❸ Rotating and to-and-fro rubbing methods: Shake the wrist and finger joints of the affected limb with the rotating method, and then rub the wrist with the rubbing method. The strength should ideally be enough to allow the heat generated to penetrate the skin.

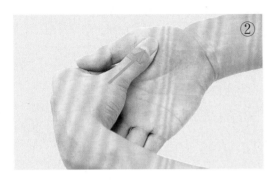 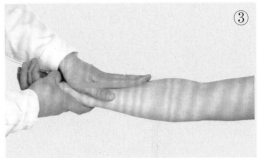

❹ Pressing method: Hold the palm of the affected limb with both hands together and press the wrist joint with a slightly heavier pressure.

❺ Rotating and finger pressing methods: Hold the affected limb with both hands and shake the wrist joint, applying a coordinated force when shaking. Press the back of the wrist with the thumb to stretch it to the maximum, then flex it and rotate the wrist 2 to 3 times on each side.

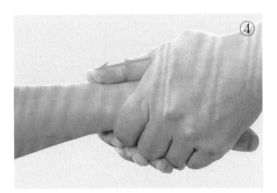 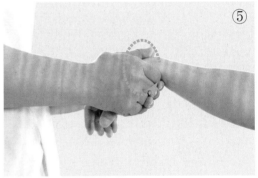

13. Wrist Sprain

A common wrist complaint is the spraining of the soft tissues around the joint. This is generally common for patients with a history of physical trauma, such as in laborious work, sport, or daily life. It can also be caused by a sudden exertion of the wrist on the ground to break a fall, and sudden rotation, extension, and flexion of the wrist joint due to holding objects. Acute injuries are characterized by painful swelling of the wrist, limited functional activity, increased pain during activity, and significant localized pressure pain. The massage techniques in this book are mainly applicable to acute wrist sprains.

Tui na duration: Approximately one minute on each acupoint.

Principles of treatment: To relax the tendons and activate blood circulation, to activate collaterals, and alleviate pain.

Steps

❶ Pressing-kneading method: With the palm side of the affected limb facing upward, press with the thumb pulp, focusing on the Neiguan and Daling acupoints, to the extent that the patient feels sore.

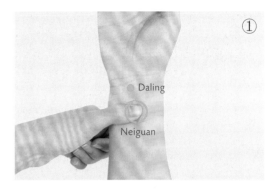

❷ Single finger meditation pushing method: Have the patient seated upright. Place a pillow or a towel under the forearm and wrist of the affected limb. Then, apply the single finger meditation pushing method around the wrist joint, especially at the pressure points, with gentle strokes.

❸ Rotating and to-and-fro rubbing methods: First shake the wrist and finger joints of the affected limb with the rotating method, and then rub the wrist with the rubbing method to relax the tendons and activate the collaterals. The movements should be slow.

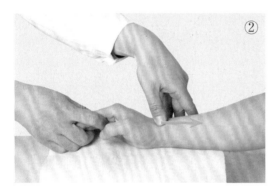

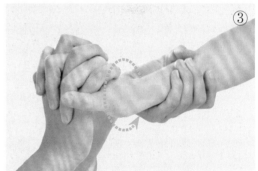

❹ Finger pressing method: With the back of the patient's hand facing upward, place the thumb on the dorsal side of the wrist joint and press the end of the thumb into the dorsal space of the wrist joint with a light and gradual force, starting from a shallow to a deep position. Ideally, this will produce soreness, numbness, and swelling.

❺ Rotating and finger pressing methods: Hold the affected limb with both hands and shake the wrist joint slowly. Then, finger press the back of the wrist with the thumb, flex to the maximum, and rotate the wrist 2 to 3 times on each side.

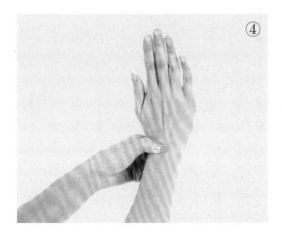

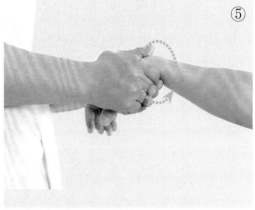

14. Tennis Elbow

The main symptom of tennis elbow is pain on the outside of the elbow, which is commonly seen in tennis players. If the wrist is repeatedly stretched (for example, when using the tennis backhand stroke), the tendons of this group of muscles may be partially strained, leading to tennis elbow.

Tui na duration: Approximately two minutes for each affected area.

Principles of treatment: To relax the tendons, dredge the collaterals, and to promote blood circulation and remove blood stasis.

Points to note: Rest the wrist and stop movements that cause elbow pain, such as playing tennis and doing housework.

Steps

❶ Rolling, grasping-kneading, and finger pressing methods: Hold the patient's arm with one hand, and with the other hand, along the lateral side of the elbow of the affected limb, apply the rolling, grasping-kneading, and pressing methods towards the upper end of the forearm, mainly to massage the pain point. Note that the speed should be even.

❷ Finger pressing and rotating methods: Place the patient's palm in an upward facing position. Place one hand on the elbow and the thumb press on the pain point; the other hand is placed on the lower end of the forearm. Rotate the forearm from inside to outside. The patient's elbow joint should be relaxed, and the practitioner's movements should be flexible and consistent.

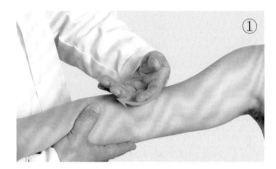
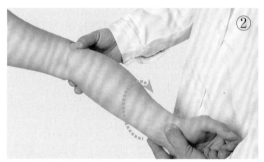

❸ Finger pressing method: Straighten the elbow of the affected limb. Place one hand on the lower end of the forearm and press the pain point with the thumb of the other hand for about two minutes. The pressure should be strong.

❹ Rotating method: Rotate the forearm of the affected limb forward, while flexing and straightening the elbow, and rotate and rock back and forth 6 to 7 times. The movement should be gentle.

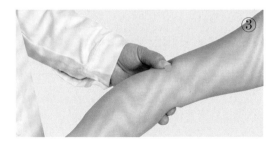
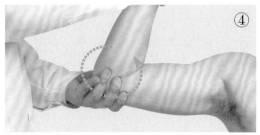

❺ Plucking method: Place the thumb on the pain point of the elbow of the affected limb. Taking the pain point as the center, pluck the area with the thumb. This should include the muscle fibers. Note that the strength should go from light to heavy.

❻ To-and-fro rubbing method: The patient's upper limb is relaxed. Taking the pain point at the elbow as the center, perform the to-and-fro rubbing method with the palm, applying even pressure.

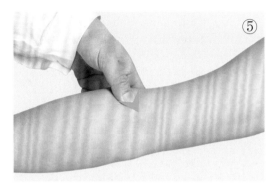
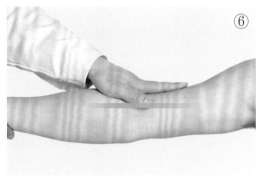

15. Knee Synovitis

Knee synovitis is an inflammation of the synovial membrane caused by irritation, resulting in an increase and accumulation of synovial fluid secretion. The knee is the joint with the most synovial membranes in the body, so synovitis is more common there.

Tui na duration: Approximately 3 to 5 minutes for each acupoint.

Principles of treatment: To relax the tendons, dredge the collaterals, and to promote blood circulation and remove blood stasis.

Points to note: Reduce the load on the knee joint and avoid excessive movement of the knee joint.

Steps

❶ Finger-pressing and kneading method: Gently finger-press and knead the pain points around the knee joint of the affected limb with the pulp of the thumb for 3 to 5 minutes. This method has the effect of relaxing the tendons and activating the blood.

❷ Pressing-kneading method: Place the pulp of thumb and index finger on the Neixiyan and Waixiyan acupoints of the affected knee respectively and gently press for 3 to 5 minutes. The patient should feel sore.

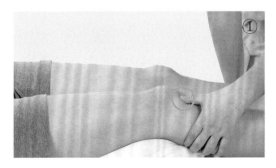
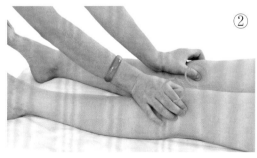

❸ Circular rubbing method: Apply the circular rubbing method to the knee joint and surrounding area using the palm for about five minutes until a warm sensation is experienced.

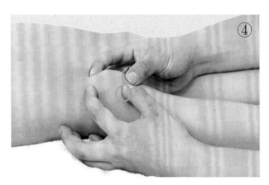

❹ Pressing-kneading method: Have the patient straighten their leg or lie in a supine position. Place the thumb and index finger of both hands on each side of the patella, and focus the thumb pulp on pressing-kneading the patella. The movement should be gentle, and the force should be steady.

❺ Stretching method: Have the patient lying on their back. Hold the calf of the affected limb and lift it up. Coordinate your arms and body when exerting force, and pull the knee joint upwards. The force applied should be even. In case of severe pain, include the circular rubbing method and apply wet hot compress.

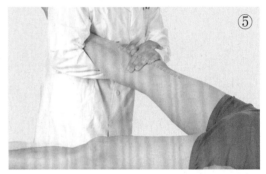

16. Hip Bursitis

The hip bursa is located around the hip tendon and joint, and contains a small amount of synovial fluid, which plays a role in reducing friction and cushioning shock. Inflammation occurs when the hip bursa is stretched and squeezed due to long-term excessive abduction of the lower limb, prolonged standing and sitting, overexertion, exposure to pathogenic wind, cold and dampness, falls, and bruises on the hip joint. Many patients only feel discomfort and soreness in the affected limb, and can still walk as usual. Discomfort during walking only occurs 2 to 3 days after the injury, and it becomes increasingly difficult to move around. The hip joint will experience pressure and pain. This pain is aggravated when joint moves, resulting in decreased hip joint mobility. There is also sound when one flexes the hip.

Tui na duration: Approximately five minutes for each part of the affected area.

Principles of treatment: To relax the tendons and promote blood circulation.

Points to note: Take good rest, try not to take the stairs and run, and do not sit on hard benches.

Steps

❶ Rolling method: Have the patient lying in a prone position, or on their side with the injured hip on the top. Apply the rolling method on the hip joint for about five minutes. The patient's lumbar area should be relaxed during the massage.

❷ To-and-fro rubbing method: Rub the lateral and anterior side of the hip joint using the palm until the heat generated penetrates the skin.

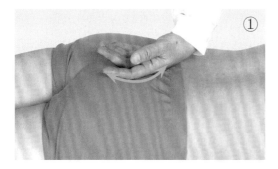
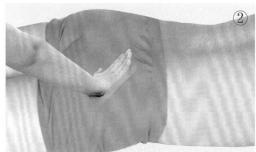

❸ Rotating method: Have the patient lying in a supine position. Hold the front side of their knee with one hand and their calf with the other. Flex the knee and hip, and then gently rock the hip joint. Then gently rotate the affected lower limb internally and flex the hip upward as much as possible. Pull the affected limb downwards and flatten it against the surface. This *tui na* method should be executed slowly.

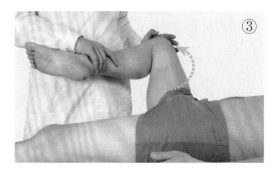

❹ Pulling-shaking method: Have the patient lying in a supine position. Hold the affected lower limb with both hands and perform antagonistic traction on the posterior side of the calf, followed by upward lifting and traction. The patient's hip joint is externally rotated and abducted and straightened under traction. The patient should ideally feel local tremors.

❺ Plucking method: Once the patient's condition is alleviated, perform the plucking method on the muscles around the hip joint to release spasms and relax the muscles.

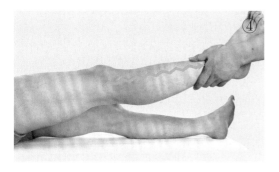
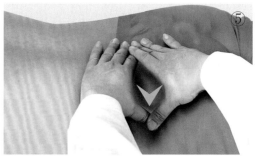

17. Achilles Tendonitis

Achilles tendonitis is an inflammation of the Achilles tendon and tendon periphery, and is a form of aseptic chronic trauma. Most cases are caused by running and jumping movements with excessive load on the lower limbs, when the ankle joint is flexed and stretched rapidly and the Achilles tendon is stretched and strained repeatedly for a long time without any obvious history of direct trauma, and the blood vessels in the muscle are stretched and squeezed to cause damage to the Achilles tendon.

Tui na duration: Approximately 2 to 5 minutes for each area.

Principles of treatment: To relax the tendons, dredge the collaterals, and to reduce swelling and alleviate pain.

Points to note: Rest the affected limb during an acute attack.

Steps

❶ Rolling method: Have the patient lying in a prone position, with the calf and ankle cushioned with a thin pillow. Apply the rolling method along the Achilles tendon to the back of the calf. This method can relieve discomfort in the Achilles tendon.

❷ Pinching-grasping method: Have the patient lying in a prone position. Hold the gastrocnemius muscle with both hands. One side is grasped and pinched for about two minutes before switching to the other side. This method can effectively relax the leg muscles.

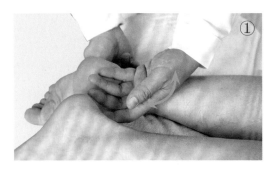
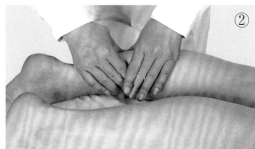

❸ Pinching method: Have the patient lying in a prone position. Stand on the patient's affected side and pinch the Achilles tendon with the thumb and other four fingers for about two minutes. Apply slightly more force when using this method.

❹ Holding twisting method: Have the patient lying in a prone position. Hold and twist the Achilles tendon with the thumb and index finger for about two minutes. This method should be executed quickly.

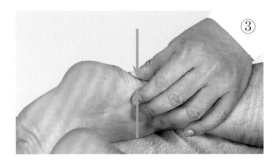
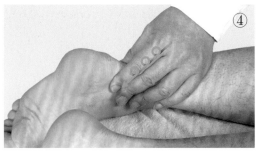

❺ Rotating method: Have the patient lying in a prone position with their knees bent at 90°. The sole should be facing up. Hold the Achilles tendon with one hand and the tip of the foot with the other. Rotate the ankle joint for about five minutes. Keep the rotation small.

❻ Pulling method: After applying the rotating method, allow some time for the muscles to relax before applying the pulling method on the ankle joint for about two minutes. Use appropriate force and do not be rough.

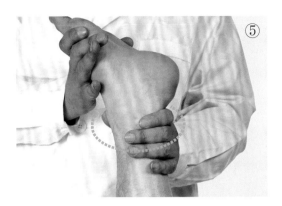
⑤

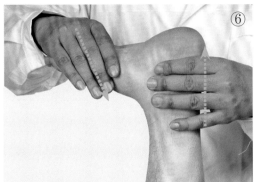
⑥

18. Ankle Sprain

An ankle sprain is an injury to the lateral ligaments of the ankle when the ankle joint is in the toe-flexion position and the ankle is turned strongly inward. It is often caused by a sudden loss of footing on uneven ground while walking or running, or a fall during cycling or soccer, which causes the foot to turn inwards excessively.

Tui na **duration:** Approximately 3 to 5 minutes for each acupoint.

Principles of treatment: To relax the tendons and promote blood circulation, and to reduce swelling and alleviate pain.

Points to note: It is advisable to apply cold compress with ice to stop the bleeding and pain at the initial post-injury stage. Perform *tui na* massage after 24 hours.

Steps

❶ Pressing-kneading method: Have the patient lying on their back. Press-knead the injured area with the thumb, spreading out to the surrounding area, and then from the posterior side of the ankle to the calf and the Yanglingquan acupoint. Press-knead a few times. Focus on the Qiuxu, Xuanzhong, and Yanglingquan acupoints. The force used to execute this method should be slightly more, and the patient should ideally feel some soreness.

❷ Single finger meditation pushing method: Apply the single finger meditation pushing method on the affected area, spreading out to the surrounding area. The pressure should be moderate and even when massaging.

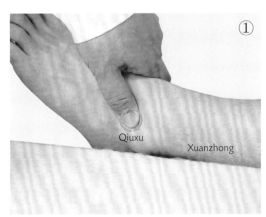
①

Qiuxu
Xuanzhong

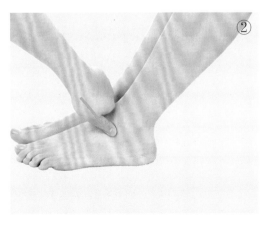
②

❸ Stretching method: Support the lower end of the patient's injured calf with one hand and hold the dorsum of the foot with the other hand. Apply a coordinated force with both arms to pull in the opposite direction and perform inversion of the ankle joint and rotate it in and out with low amplitude.

❹ Stretching and pressing-kneading methods: Hold the patient's injured foot with both hands. Gently stretch and perform eversion of the ankle joint, and apply soft pressing and kneading on the sprained area, along with internal and external rotation of the ankle joint.

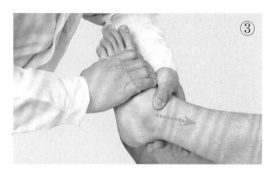
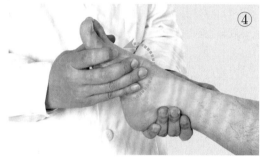

❺ Pressing-kneading and stretching methods: Gently press-knead the ankle joint with the thumb. Hold the heel of the foot with one hand, hold the back of the foot with the other hand and apply the stretching method to stretch the meridians of the foot. Note that the pressure should be even when massaging.

❻ Circular rubbing, pushing, and to-and-fro rubbing methods: Use both hands to rub the ankle several times until the skin is warm. Next, apply the pushing and to-and-fro rubbing methods on the back of the foot, through the ankle to the calf, so as to warm up the affected area.

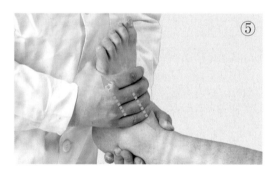
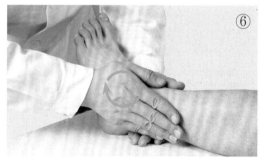

19. Heel Pain

Heel pain is a condition caused by chronic strain around the heel nodes, with pain and difficulty walking as the main symptoms. The pain is severe in the morning when getting out of bed and starting to stand or walk, and is relieved after activity. However, it can be aggravated after prolonged standing and walking, and is relieved after rest.

Tui na duration: Approximately 2 to 5 minutes for each affected area.

Principles of treatment: To relax the tendons, dredge the collaterals, and to activate blood circulation and alleviate pain.

Points to note: Patients should rest properly during the acute phase, reduce weight bearing, and should not do strenuous exercise. Pay attention to local warmth and avoid cold stimulation.

Steps

❶ Rolling method: Apply the rolling method from the injured heel to the metatarsal tendon membrane back and forth for about five minutes. This can relieve heel pain.

❷ Finger pressing method: Hold the patient's ankle with one hand and press the pain point on the heel with the thumb of the other hand for about two minutes. The pressure should be gentle, going from light to heavy.

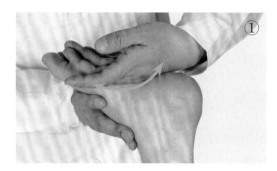 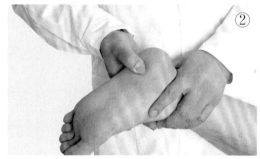

❸ Pressing-kneading method: Use one hand to hold the heel, with the thumb of the other hand pressing slightly hard on the Yangquan acupoint, to produce soreness.

❹ Pressing-kneading method: Press-knead the patient's feet with the thumb pulp in a clockwise direction for 3 to 5 minutes at the Taixi, Zhaohai and Ran'gu acupoints respectively to produce soreness.

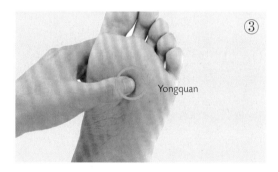 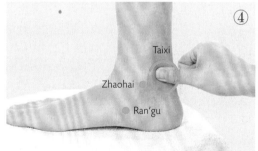

❺ Pressing-kneading method: Press-knead the patient's feet with the thumb pulp on the Kunlun and Pucan acupoints with a gradually increasing force for 3 to 5 minutes each to produce soreness.

❻ Striking method: Have the patient lying in a prone position with their knee bent at 90° and the sole of their foot facing upward. Hold the foot with one hand to support the ankle joint, and with the other

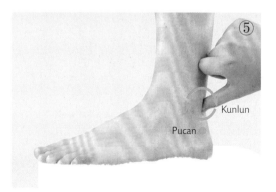

hand, strike the heel bone with a fist a few dozen times with moderate force.

❼ To-and-fro rubbing method: Keeping the patient in the same position, apply the to-and-fro rubbing method along the metatarsal tendon membrane, until the heat generated penetrates the skin.

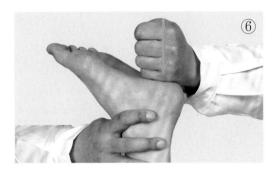

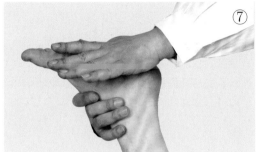

20. Knee Pain

There are many causes of knee pain. In daily life, most knee pain is not caused by trauma, but by prolonged cold and extreme temperature differences. Especially during autumn, when cold and warm temperatures alternate, low temperatures or drastic temperature differences can cause the muscles and blood vessels around the knee to contract, causing pain.

Tui na **duration:** Approximately two minutes for each affected part.

Principles of treatment: To relax the tendons, dredge the collaterals, and to promote blood circulation and remove blood stasis.

Points to note: Reduce the load on the knee joint and avoid excessive exercise of the knee joint.

Steps

❶ Finger pressing method: Have the patient lying in a supine position. Press both thumbs on the Neixiyan and Waixiyan acupoints of the affected knee with a slight force for about one minute each, to the extent where the joints feel slightly sore.

❷ Finger-pressing and kneading method: Have the patient lying in a prone position. Apply finger-pressing and kneading method using the thumb on the Weizhong acupoint of the affected knee, for about 20 to 40 times, with a gradual increase in the force applied. The amplitude of the kneading should be moderate.

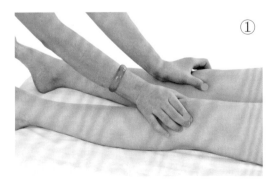

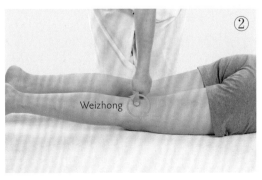

Weizhong

❸ Finger pressing method: The patient bends the knee. Apply finger pressing method with the thumb pulp on the Ququan acupoint for 30 times, with a gradual increase in the force applied.

❹ Finger pressing method: Press on the Xuehai and Liangqiu acupoints until the treatment area feels slightly sore.

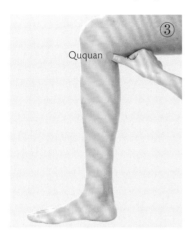
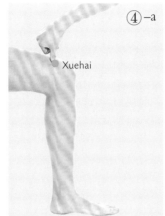
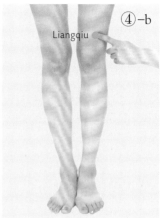

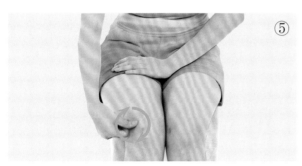

❺ Finger-pressing and kneading method: Finger-press and knead the area around the pain point with the thumb pulp. The force applied for the pressing and kneading should be moderate, and the *tui na* massage should ideally make the area feel slightly sore.

21. Rheumatic Arthritis

Rheumatic arthritis is a common acute or chronic inflammatory ailment of the connective tissue. What is commonly referred to as rheumatic arthritis is one of the main symptoms of rheumatic fever, and is clinically characterized by wandering joint and muscle soreness, redness, swelling, and pain.

Tui na duration: Approximately 1 to 3 minutes for each acupoint.

Principles of treatment: To relax the tendons, dredge the collaterals, and to promote blood circulation and remove blood stasis.

Points to note: Avoid dark and humid environments.

Steps
❶ Pressing-kneading method: Apply the pressing-kneading method with the pulp of thumb or index finger on the Yanglingquan, Zusanli, Xuehai, Liangqiu, Heding, Waixiyan and Neixiyan acupoints for 1 to 3 minutes each. The pressure applied can be slightly heavier. It is ideal to keep the patient warm and comfortable during the *tui na* massage.

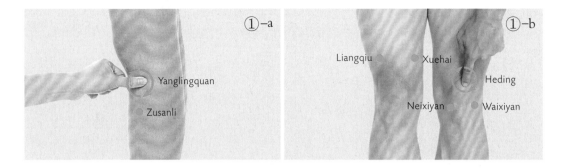

❷ Pressing-kneading method: Apply the pressing-kneading method with the pulp of thumb or index finger. Press-knead in a clockwise direction on the Jiexi, Qiuxu, Yangjiao, Kunlun, Taixi, and Xuanzhong acupoints for 1 to 3 minutes each. Local soreness should ideally be felt.

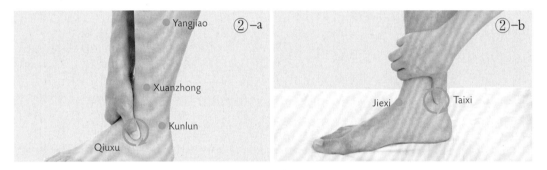

❸ Finger pressing method: Apply the finger pressing method with the pulp of thumb or index finger on the Jianliao, Jianyu, Jianjing, and Jianzhen acupoints for 1 to 3 minutes each.

❹ Pressing-kneading method: Apply the pressing-kneading method with the pulp of thumb or index finger. Press-knead in a clockwise direction on the Daling, Wan'gu, Hegu, Yangchi, Yangxi, and Waiguan acupoints for 1 to 3 minutes each.

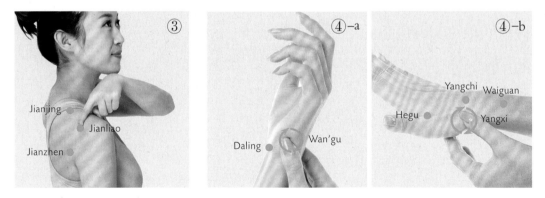

❺ Pressing-kneading method: Apply the pressing-kneading method with the pulp of thumb on the Xiaohai, Quchi, Shousanli, and Tianjing acupoints for 1 to 3 minutes each. There should ideally be local soreness. Pressing and kneading the Quchi and Shousanli acupoints can help alleviate discomfort of the elbow joint. Stimulating the Tianjing acupoint can help move *qi* and disperse knots.

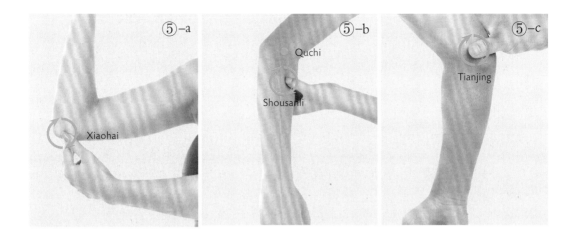

⑤-a Xiaohai

⑤-b Quchi Shousanli

⑤-c Tianjing

22. Rheumatoid Arthritis

Rheumatoid arthritis is a chronic systemic autoimmune disease with joint lesions. The main clinical symptoms are joint swelling and pain caused by the synovial membrane of small joints, followed by cartilage destruction, and narrowing of the joint space. In the advanced stages there can be severe bone destruction and resorption leading to joint stiffness, deformity, and functional impairment.

Tui na duration: Approximately 5 to 8 minutes for each affected part, two minutes on each acupoint.

Principles of treatment: To relax the tendons, dredge the collaterals, and to promote blood circulation and remove blood stasis.

Points to note: Keep your living environment dry and clean, and avoid living and working in humid conditions.

Steps

❶ Rolling method: Apply the rolling method around the affected area. The frequency of rolling should ideally be around 120 to 160 times per minute. The length of this *tui na* massage should be around eight minutes long, and passive joint exercises should be incorporated.

❷ Pressing-kneading and grasping methods: Press-knead the acupoints around the affected joint with the thumb pulp for about two minutes each. Apply the grasping method on the affected joint for about five minutes.

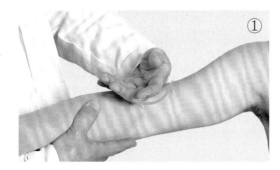

①

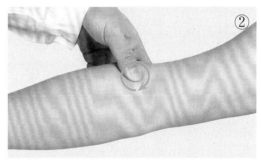

②

❸ Palm twisting, holding twisting, and rotating methods: For larger joints that are affected, apply the palm twisting method for about five minutes; for the smaller joints, apply the holding twisting method for about two minutes; for dysfunctional joints, apply the rotating method for about two minutes. The twisting should be gentle.

❹ Finger pressing method: Apply the finger pressing method with the thumb on the patient's Zhishi acupoint for 1 to 2 minutes. The pressure applied should be heavier, and it should ideally create soreness.

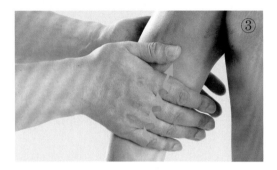
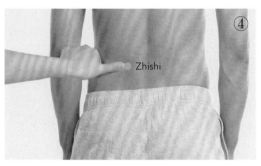

❺ Finger pressing method: Apply the finger pressing method with the thumb pulp and press in a clockwise direction on the Sanyinjiao acupoint and Taixi acupoint for about 1 to 2 minutes each. The pressure should be kept light.

❻ To-and-fro rubbing and patting methods: First apply to-and-fro rubbing on the affected joint, then apply patting method to allow the heat generated to penetrate the joint.

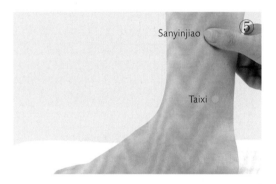
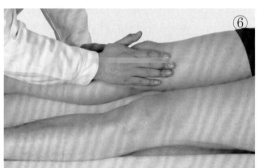

23. Acute Gouty Arthritis

Acute gouty arthritis is one of the common rheumatic diseases. It often occurs late at night with progressively increasingly unbearable joint pain like being torn, cut or bit. Some patients may have systemic symptoms such as fever, chills, headaches, palpitations, and nausea.

Tui na duration: 8 to 10 minutes on larger affected joints, 5 to 8 minutes for smaller affected joints.

Principles of treatment: To relax the tendons, dredge the collaterals, and to activate blood circulation and alleviate pain.

Points to note: When arthritis occurs, apply a hot towel to the affected area for 20 minutes every day to relieve pain.

Steps

❶ Rolling method: Apply the rolling method on the joints of all the limbs, paying attention to the affected joint. The length of this *tui na* massage should be around ten minutes, and joint functional exercises should be incorporated. This method has the effect of relaxing the tendons and promoting blood circulation, relieving spasms and pain.

❷ Single finger meditation pushing, finger pressing, and pinching-grasping methods: For smaller affected joints, use the single finger meditation pushing method for 5 to 8 minutes. Then use the pulp of thumb or middle finger to press the acupoints around the affected joint for about one minute each. Next, apply the pinching-grasping method around the affected joints for 8 to 10 minutes. The strength and frequency of the massage should be even.

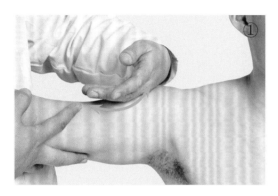
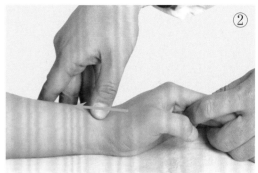

❸ Palm twisting and holding twisting methods: Apply the palm twisting method on larger joints that are affected, for about 8 to 10 minutes. Apply the holding twisting method on affected smaller joints for about 5 to 8 minutes. Note that the area that is being massaged should be relaxed.

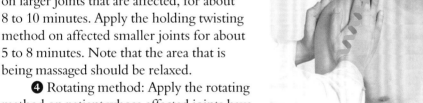

❹ Rotating method: Apply the rotating method on patient whose affected joints have limited their mobility. The length of the *tui na* massage should be around five minutes, and the massage should be gentle.

❺ To-and-fro rubbing and pulling-shaking methods: Apply the to-and-fro rubbing method on the affected joint until the heat generated penetrates into the skin. Then, complete the session with the pulling-shaking method.

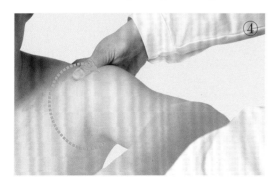
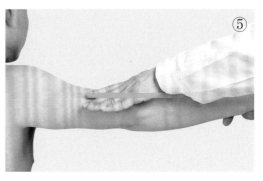

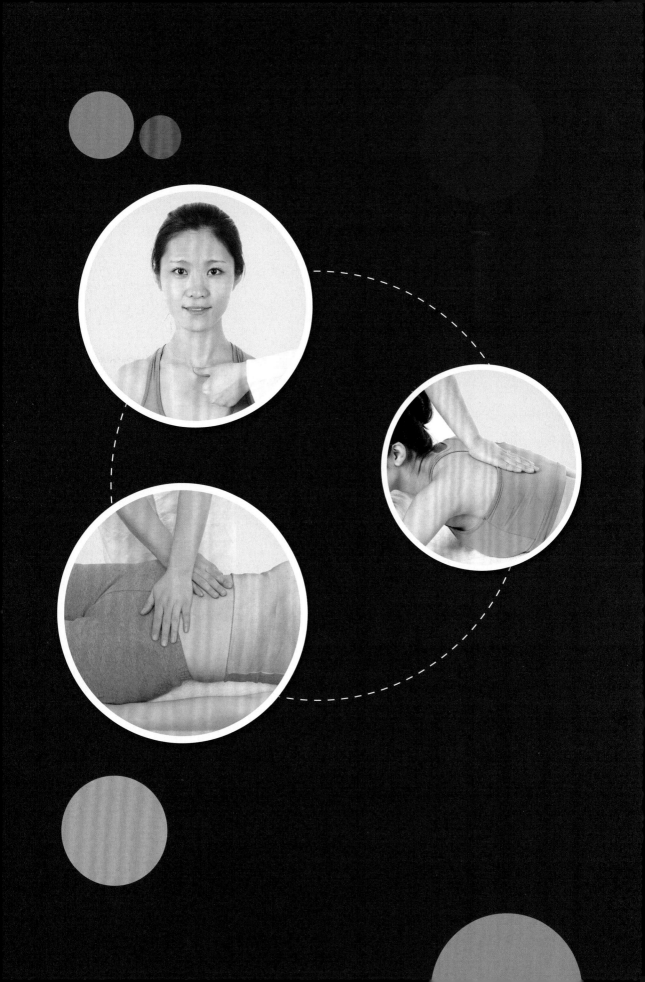

CHAPTER THREE
Relieving Internal Diseases through *Tui Na*

Colds, coughs, and constipation are ailments that almost everyone encounters. Although they are not major problems, they can be inconvenient. Symptoms of these common minor ailments can be relieved through *tui na*. Pick up some *tui na* methods, and when you feel uncomfortable, you can relieve the discomfort through *tui na* massage.

Note: Due to the angle of the pictures, not all of the acupoints are marked in some pictures in the text. See the appendix for common *tui na* acupoints. When massaging, you can either complete all the steps, or you can select some of the steps according to your own situation. Massage both acupoints if they are symmetrically distributed on the body.

1. Cold

A cold is a common illness caused by external pathogenic wind, and can manifest as nasal congestion, a runny nose, sneezing, coughing, headaches, chills, fever, and general bodily discomfort. It can occur all year round, but especially in winter and spring. According to the various causes and symptoms, colds can be divided into wind-cold, wind-heat, summer-heat dampness, and *qi*-deficiency types.

Wind-cold type: Heavy cold, light fever, no sweating, headache, aching limbs, heavy nasal congestion, sometimes a runny nose, itchy throat, coughing, thin and white phlegm, no thirst or craving for hot drinks, thin white and moist tongue coating.

Wind-heat type: Fever, slight aversion to wind, non-physiological sweating or non-sweating, head swelling and pain, cough, sticky or yellow phlegm, dry throat or red, swollen, painful throat, stuffy nose, yellow runny nose, thirsty, thin yellow tongue coating, red tongue edge.

Summer-heat dampness type: Fever, slight aversion to wind, sweating (which does not relieve the fever), stuffy and runny nose, dizziness and heavy swelling, a heavy feeling and lethargy, thirst, chest tightness and vomiting, limited yellowish urine, red tongue with a greasy yellowish coating.

***Qi*-deficiency type:** Aversion to cold, fever without sweating, headache, body aches, cough with white phlegm, tiredness and weakness, aversion to wind and easy sweating, fatigue, recurrent susceptibility to the slightest inadvertence, light, thin white coating on the tongue.

Basic Steps

❶ Pushing and finger-pressing and kneading methods: Apply the pushing method using the thumb pulp on the Yintang acupoint 8 to 10 times, followed by gently finger-pressing and kneading on both sides of the Taiyang, Cuanzhu, and Yingxiang acupoints for one minute each. Next, push the forehead, upper and lower orbits, and both sides of the nose 5 to 8 times. The force applied should be moderate.

❷ Grasping method: Apply the grasping method on the Fengchi acupoints using the thumb and index finger, followed by slowly moving down to the sides of the neck. Repeat this motion 8 to 10 times. Next, apply the five-finger grasping method from the front of the hairline to the back of the hairline 5 to 8 times. This method has the effect of unblocking meridians.

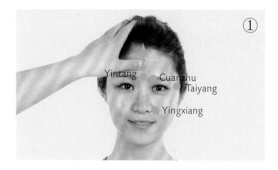
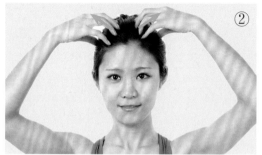

❸ To-and-fro rubbing method: Have the patient lying in a prone position. Apply to-and-fro rubbing along the Dazhui acupoint and Taiyang Bladder Meridian of Foot on the upper back with hypothenar, to the extent that the heat generated penetrates the skin.

❹ Grasping method: Have the patient lying in a prone position. Hold Jianjing acupoints on both sides of the shoulder with the thumb and other four fingers. Apply the grasping method with slight pressure to generate soreness.

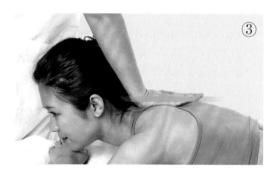
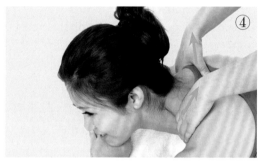

Additional Steps for the Wind-Cold Type

❶ Kneading method: Use the thumb pulp to knead the Feishu and Fengmen acupoints in a clockwise direction. The *tui na* massage should not be too forceful, and should ideally generate soreness.

❷ Finger-pressing and kneading method: Apply the finger-pressing and kneading

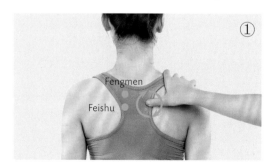
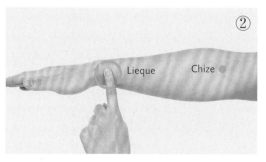

method with the thumb or index finger on the patient's Lieque and Chize acupoints. The *tui na* massage can be slightly forceful and should ideally generate soreness, numbness, and bloating.

Additional Steps for the Wind-Heat Type

❶ Kneading method: Apply the kneading method using the thumb pulp, and knead the Zhongfu and Yunmen acupoints for 1 to 2 minutes each. The *tui na* massage should ideally generate soreness and the movement should be gentle.

❷ Finger-pressing and kneading method: Apply the finger-pressing and kneading method using the thumb pulp on the patient's Quchi, Hegu, and Waiguan acupoints for one minute each. The force of the *tui na* massage should gradually increase and should ideally generate soreness, numbness, and bloating.

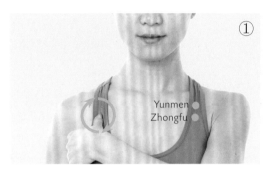
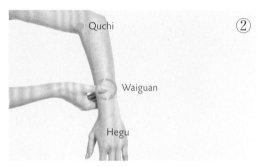

Additional Steps for the Summer-Heat Dampness Type

❶ Kneading and circular rubbing methods: Apply the kneading method using the thumb pulp, and knead the Zhongwan and Tianshu acupoints with moderate force until soreness is generated. Then supplement with the circular rubbing method on the abdomen in a clockwise direction.

❷ Finger-pressing and kneading method: Apply finger-pressing and kneading method using the thumb on the patient's Fengchi and Jianjing acupoints to generate soreness, numbness, and bloating. Knead the acupoints on both sides at the same time.

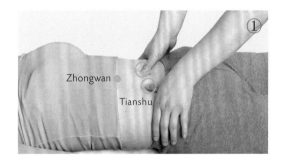
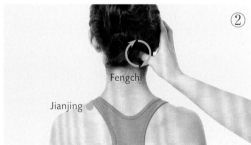

Additional Steps for the *Qi*-Deficiency Type

❶ Kneading method: Have the patient lying in a supine position. Gently knead the Qihai and Guanyuan acupoints with the thumb for one minute each, until soreness is generated.

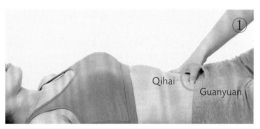

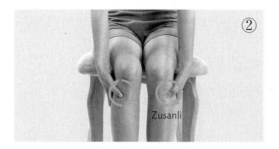

Zusanli

❷ Kneading method: Have the patient seated upright. Knead both sides of the patient's Zusanli acupoints with the thumb pulps of both hands simultaneously to generate soreness and bloating.

2. Cough

The causes of coughing can be classified as externally infected or arising from endogenous injuries. Wind-cold coughs and wind-heat coughs are caused by external infection, while coughs with phlegm-damp amassing in lung and coughs with liver fire invading lung are mainly caused by endogenous injuries. The symptoms of a cough will vary with the causes.

Wind-cold cough: A heavy cough with thin white phlegm, accompanied by headache and a stiff neck, stuffy nose, clear nasal mucus, aching bone joints, aversion to cold, no sweating or other superficies syndromes, pale tongue with a thin white coating.

Wind-heat cough: A cough with thick breath, thick yellow phlegm, sweating and thirst, a sore throat, usually accompanied by superficies syndromes such as nasal congestion, yellow nasal mucus, aversion to wind and fever, with thin yellow tongue coating.

Coughs with phlegm-damp amassing in lung: A recurrent cough, heavy coughing, lots of sticky or thick lumpy phlegm, grayish white phlegm, coughing in the morning or after eating, and coughing with phlegm which is aggravated by eating sweet and oily food, accompanied by anorexia, fatigue, loose stool, and a greasy white tongue coating.

Coughs with liver fire invading lung: Cough with dyspnea, red face and pain in the two hypochondrium when coughing, often feeling that phlegm is stuck in the throat and is difficult to get out, with low quantity and a sticky quality, accompanied by distension and pain in the chest and hypochondrium, and a dry and bitter mouth; symptoms may increase or decrease due to mood swings, with a red tongue and limited saliva.

Basic Steps

❶ Pressing-kneading method: Apply the pressing-kneading method with the thumb pulp, pressing on the Tiantu, Danzhong, Qihu, and Wuyi acupoints for one minute each with moderate force until the patient feels sore.

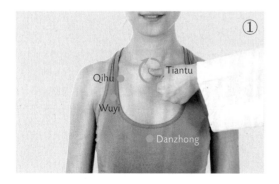

Qihu · Tiantu · Wuyi · Danzhong

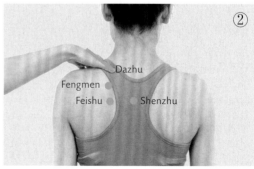

Dazhu · Fengmen · Feishu · Shenzhu

❷ Single finger meditation pushing method: Apply the single finger meditation pushing method on the Dazhu, Shenzhu, Fengmen, and Feishu acupoints for one minute each. More force can be applied, ideally to generate soreness.

❸ Single finger meditation pushing method: Apply the single finger meditation pushing method on the Chize and Taiyuan acupoints for 2 to 3 minutes each. The force applied should gradually increase, ideally to generate soreness, numbness, and bloating.

❹ Pressing-kneading method: Apply the pressing-kneading method with the thumb pulp, and massage the Lieque, Waiguan, and Hegu acupoints for 1 to 2 minutes each, ideally to generate soreness.

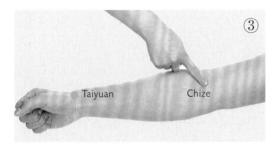
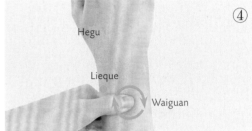

Additional Steps for Wind-Cold Cough

❶ Kneading method: Apply the kneading method using the thumb pulp on the Fengchi and Fengfu acupoints for one minute each. The force applied should be moderate and should ideally generate soreness.

❷ Kneading and to-and-fro rubbing methods: Have the patient lying in a prone position. Knead and to-and-fro rub along the two sides of the Taiyang Bladder Meridian of Foot on the back until the skin feels warm.

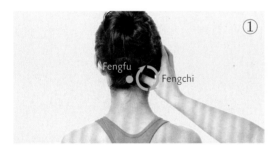
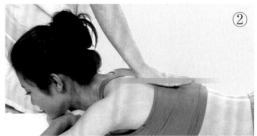

Additional Steps for Wind-Heat Cough

❶ Kneading method: Apply the kneading method using the thumb pulp, and knead the Zhongfu and Yunmen acupoints for one minute each, until the patient feels sore. This

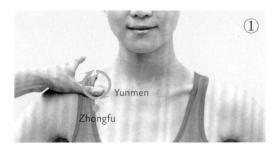
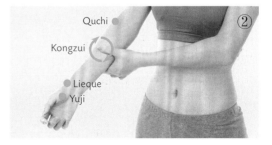

method can also be executed with the patient lying in a prone position.

❷ Finger-pressing and kneading method: Finger-press and knead the Quchi, Kongzui, Lieque, and Yuji acupoints for one minute each, ideally to generate soreness, numbness, and bloating.

Additional Steps for Coughs with Phlegm-Damp Amassing in Lung
❶ Single finger meditation pushing method: Have the patient lying in a supine position. Apply the single finger meditation pushing method on the Zhongwan, Tianshu, Qihai, and Guanyuan acupoints for 1 to 2 minutes each. The force of the *tui na* massage should be light, ideally to generate soreness.

❷ Finger pressing and to-and-fro rubbing methods: Finger press on the Pishu, Weishu, and Shenshu acupoints for one minute each, ideally to generate soreness and bloating. Supplement with transversely to-and-fro rubbing on the lumbosacral region to activate heat penetration.

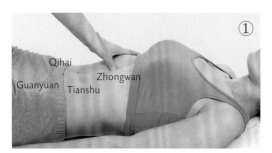
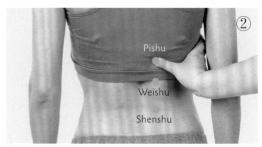

Additional Steps for Coughs with Liver Fire Invading Lung
❶ Kneading method: Have the patient seated upright. Apply the kneading method on the Xinshu and Ganshu acupoints for 2 to 3 minutes each, until the patient feels sore. As the back is meaty and thick, this method should be executed with more force.

❷ Pushing and finger-pressing and kneading methods: Have the patient lying in a supine position. Push the two hypochondrium from the Conception Vessel along the rib cage with two thumbs, from inside out 5 to 10 times. Then press and knead the Qimen and Zhangmen acupoints with the thumb for 1 to 2 minutes each, until the patient feels sore.

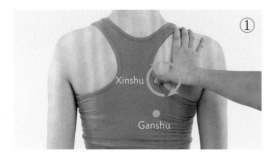
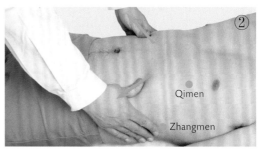

3. Asthma

Asthma is a common recurring ailment. Croup and wheezing are both types of shortness of breath, but they differ in symptoms. For croup, the symptoms are shortness of breath with a wheezing sound or even wheezing and unable to lie down. The symptoms of wheezing include shortness of breath and even with mouth open and shoulder lifted, flaring of nose wing, and inability to lie down.

Externally assaulted wind-cold asthma: Wheezing and coughing with shortness of breath, a whistling sound in the throat, stuffy chest, thin and white sputum, headache, aversion to cold, or fever, no thirst, no sweating, thin white and smooth tongue coating.

Externally assaulted wind-heat asthma: Wheezing and coughing, phlegm in the throat sounding like roaring, chest tightness and bloating, coughing and choking, sticky and yellow or blood-colored phlegm, higher body temperature, sweating, red face, bitter mouth, dry throat, thirst, red tongue, yellow and greasy tongue coating.

Asthma with turbid phlegm: Asthma and cough, phlegm that is sticky and unpleasant to cough up, a phlegmy sound in the throat, chest tightness, nausea and anorexia, a bland taste in the mouth, greasy white tongue coating.

Lung and kidney *yin*-deficiency asthma: Shallow breathing, shortness of breath especially when moving, weight loss and fatigue, sweating and cold limbs, light tongue with red coating.

Basic Steps

❶ Pushing method: Apply the pushing method on one side of the Qiaogong acupoint from top to bottom 20 to 30 times, then repeat on the other side. Push from the forehead to the lower jaw. Repeat 2 to 3 times.

❷ Grasping and grasping-kneading methods: Apply the grasping method from the patient's head to the occipital area with five fingers, and from the occipital area to the neck with three fingers. Repeat this 3 to 4 times. Next, grasp-knead the Fengchi and Jianjing acupoints for 1 to 2 minutes, ideally producing soreness.

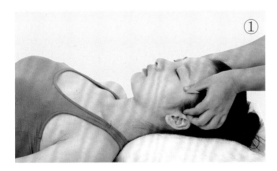
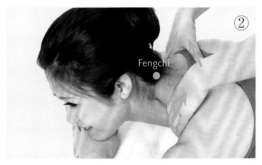

❸ Single finger meditation pushing and to-and-fro rubbing methods: Apply the single finger meditation pushing method from the patient's Tiantu acupoint to Shenque acupoint.

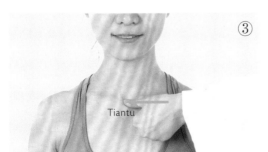
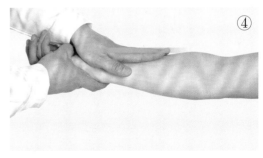

Focus on the Tiantu and Danzhong acupoints. Then use the palm to transversely rub to-and-fro on the chest, starting from the inferior margin of clavicle to the twelfth rib. Repeat this 2 to 3 times, ideally producing soreness.

❹ To-and-fro rubbing and grasping methods: Rub the inner side of the arm with the palm of the hand until the heat generated penetrates the skin, and then grasp from the shoulder to the wrist. Apply this on one side first, then switch to the other side.

Additional Steps for Externally Assaulted Wind-Cold Asthma

❶ Kneading method: Apply the kneading method using the thumb pulp, and knead the Fengmen, Feishu, and Dingchuan acupoints. This should ideally generate soreness.

❷ To-and-fro rubbing and finger-pressing and kneading methods: Rub along the Taiyang Bladder Meridian of Foot on the upper back until the skin feels warm. Next, finger-press and knead with the thumb on the Dazhui, Fengchi, Jianjing, Jianzhongshu and Jianwaishu acupoints for one minute each, until soreness is generated.

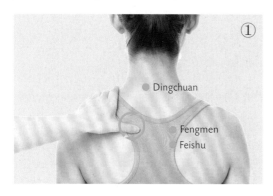
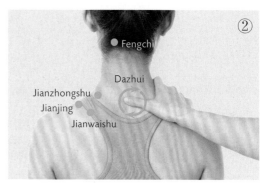

Additional Steps for Externally Assaulted Wind-Heat Asthma

❶ Single finger meditation pushing and pushing methods: Apply the single finger meditation pushing method, pushing the patient's Tiantu, Danzhong, Quepen, Qihu, and Wuyi acupoints for 1 to 2 minutes each, until soreness is produced. This is supplemented by pushing on the Conception Vessel (the Conception Vessel runs in the middle line of the abdomen. Pressing from the naval down to three cun below the umbilicus helps to unblock the Conception Vessel) and the two sides of the rib, until warmth is felt. This method can also be performed with the patient lying in a supine position.

❷ Pressing-kneading method: Press the patient's Quchi, Lieque, and Chize acupoints for one minute each with moderate force until soreness is generated.

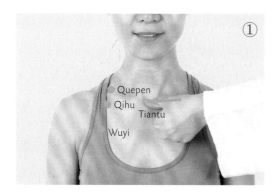
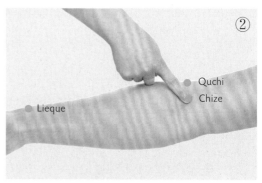

Additional Steps for Asthma with Turbid Phlegm

❶ Finger-pressing and kneading method: Have the patient lying in a supine position, or in a comfortable position. Finger-press and knead the Pishu acupoint with the thumb pulp in a clockwise direction.

❷ Finger-pressing and kneading method: Press and knead the patient's Xuehai, Yinlingquan, Sanyinjiao, Zusanli, and Fenglong acupoints with thumb pulp until soreness is generated.

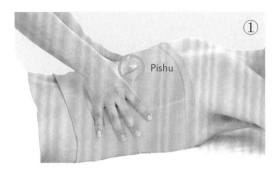
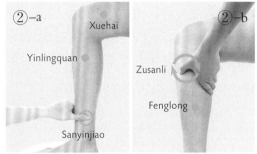

Additional Steps for Lung and Kidney *Yin*-Deficiency Asthma

❶ Kneading and to-and-fro rubbing methods: Knead the Shenshu and Pishu acupoints with the thumb pulp, then to-and-fro rub the Baliao acupoints, until warmth is felt. This method can also be applied to the patient lying in a supine position.

❷ Single finger meditation pushing and vibrating methods: First push the patient's Qihai and Guanyuan acupoints, then use the vibrating method with the palm on the Guanyuan acupoint until the heat generated penetrates the lumbosacral area and warmth is felt.

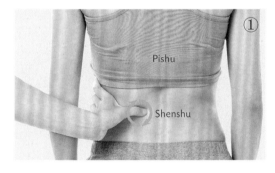
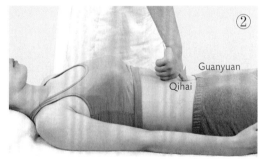

4. Diarrhea

Diarrhea refers to an increase in the number of bowel movements, thin stools, or even watery discharge. It is characterized by either thin stools with slow discharge or watery stools that discharge quickly. It is an ailment that can occur throughout the year, although it is more commonly seen during summer and autumn.

Damp-heat type diarrhea: Diarrhea with abdominal pain, quick or inadequate diarrhea, yellowish-brown facial color with a foul odor, burning sensation on the anus, irritable mood with thirst, limited yellow urine, red tongue with a greasy yellow coating.

Damp-cold type diarrhea: Clear and diluted diarrhea, sometimes resembling water, bloated stomach with poor appetite, abdominal pain and borborygmus. If combined with external wind-cold, then there will be symptoms such as cold, fever, headache, aching limbs, and a white or greasy tongue coating.

Deficiency of spleen and stomach type diarrhea: Occasional loose stools and diarrhea with high recurrence, lack of appetite, and a bloated feeling after eating. If slightly greasy food is consumed, the frequency of toilet runs will increase significantly, sallow complexion, fatigue and a light tongue color with white coating.

Liver *qi* invading spleen type diarrhea: This type of diarrhea is triggered by emotional factors and mood swings. Usually there is abdominal pain and borborygmus, fullness and discomfort in chest and hypochondrium belch and lack of appetite, and a thin coating on the tongue.

Basic Steps

❶ Single finger meditation pushing method: Have the patient lying in a supine position. Apply a slow and steady single finger meditation pushing method from the Zhongwan acupoint down to the Qihai and Guanyuan acupoints. Repeat this motion 5 to 6 times, and be gentle.

❷ Circular rubbing method: Apply the circular rubbing method with the palm on the stomach in an anti-clockwise motion for 3 to 5 minutes.

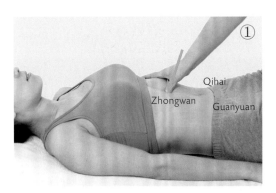
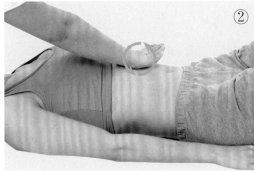

❸ Rolling method: Have the patient lying in a prone position. Apply the rolling method along both sides of the spine, from the Pishu to the Dachangshu acupoints with slightly more force. Repeat 5 to 6 times.

❹ Pressing-kneading method: Press-knead the Weishu and Changqiang acupoints with the thumb pulp for 1 to 2 minutes each.

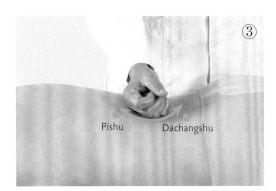
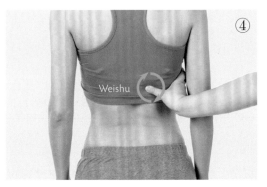

Additional Steps for Damp-Heat Type Diarrhea

❶ Pressing-kneading method: Have the patient lying in a prone position. Apply the pressing-kneading method on the patient's Ganshu and Danshu acupoints with the thumb pulp. More force should be applied for the *tui na* massage, ideally to create soreness.

❷ Circular rubbing and finger pressing methods: Apply the circular rubbing method on the stomach using the palm for about five minutes, ideally until growling noises can be heard and diarrhoea is induced. This helps to expel dampness and stop diarrhoea. Next, use the thumb pulp to press the Neiguan acupoint with moderate force.

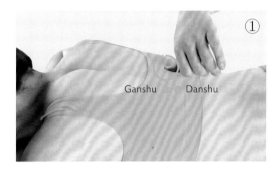
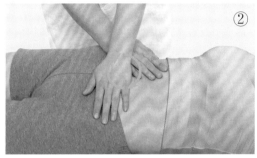

Additional Steps for Damp-Cold Type Diarrhea

❶ To-and-fro rubbing method: Have the patient lying in a prone position. Apply the to-and-fro rubbing method with the palm on the patient's Xuanshu, Mingmen, and Baliao acupoints to generate heat to the stomach.

❷ Grasping and finger-pressing and kneading methods: Apply a grasping method on the neck and the Taiyang Bladder Meridian of Foot along the shoulder and back, then finger-press and knead the Fengchi and Jianjing acupoints for 1 to 2 minutes each. Slightly more force should be applied, ideally to generate soreness.

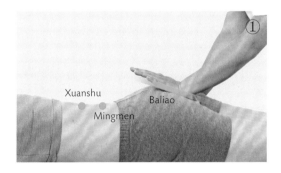
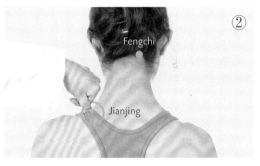

Additional Steps for Deficiency of Spleen and Stomach Type Diarrhea

❶ Pinching method: Have the patient lying in a prone position. Apply the pinching method on the patient's back. Lift and push the skin upwards once every three pinches. The force applied with the pinching should be moderate.

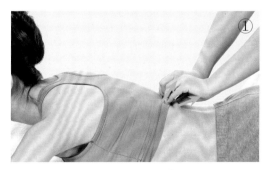

❷ Pressing method: Have the patient lying in a supine position. Stack both hands on top of one another and press on the Shenque acupoint with the palm repeatedly and rhythmically for 2 to 5 minutes, until the heat generated penetrates the skin.

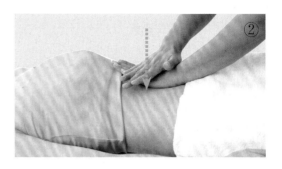

Additional Steps for Liver *Qi* Invading Spleen Type Diarrhea

❶ Kneading method: Have the patient lying in a prone position. Apply the kneading method with the thumb pulp on the patient's Ganshu, Danshu, Pishu and Weishu acupoints for 1 to 2 minutes each, until there is soreness.

❷ Finger pressing method: Have the patient lying in a supine position. Press on the Qimen and Zhangmen acupoints. Push the two hypochondrium from the Conception Vessel along the rib cage.

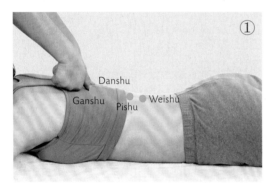

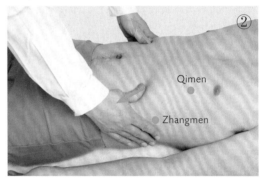

5. Vomiting

Vomiting is a condition caused by the failure of stomach *qi* to descend and the reverse flow of *qi*, and can occur in many ailments. Treatment is based on the principle of harmonizing the stomach and lowering adverse *qi*, but should be handled separately according to the various conditions and deficiencies.

Vomiting caused by external pathogens: Sudden vomiting, fullness in the chest and epigastrium, fever and aversion to cold, head and body pain, greasy white tongue coating, or a record of being invaded by external cold, heat, or dampness.

Vomiting caused by food stagnation: Eating disorders, vomiting and acid reflux, distention and fullness in the abdomen, belching and anorexia, extreme stool condition, poor bowel movement, thick and greasy tongue coating.

Vomiting with liver *qi* invading stomach: Vomiting and acid reflux, frequent belching, distension and pain in the chest and hypochondrium, red tongue with white greasy coating.

Vomiting caused by spleen and stomach *qi* deficiency: Loss of appetite, indigestion, nausea and vomiting, stuffiness in the stomach and epigastrium, irregular stools, greasy white tongue coating.

Basic Steps

❶ Single finger meditation pushing and circular rubbing methods: Have the patient lying in a supine position. Use a light and fast single finger meditation pushing method along the abdominal Conception Vessel from top to bottom, focusing on the Zhongwan acupoint for about five minutes. Then, apply the circular rubbing method with the palm on the upper abdomen for 2 to 3 minutes.

❷ Finger pressing method: Use the thumb pulp to press on the patient's Tianshu and Shenque acupoints for 2 to 3 minutes each, until soreness is generated.

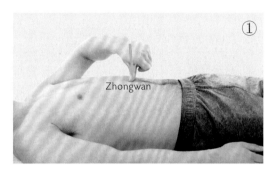
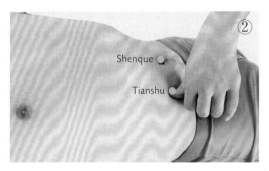

❸ Single finger meditation pushing method: Have the patient lying in a prone position. Press on both sides of the Taiyang Bladder Meridian of Foot on the back from top to bottom 5 to 8 times, until soreness is generated.

❹ Finger-pressing and kneading method: Have the patient seated upright. Press and knead the Geshu, Pishu, and Weishu acupoints using the pulp of index finger, in a clockwise direction for 2 to 3 minutes each, until soreness is generated.

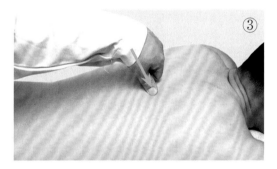
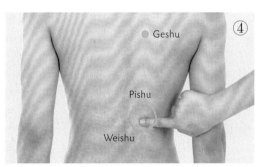

Additional Steps for Vomiting Caused by External Pathogens

❶ Finger pressing method: Press on the Neiguan and Hegu acupoints using the thumb pulp

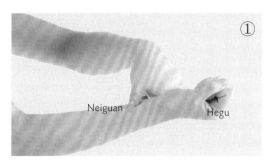
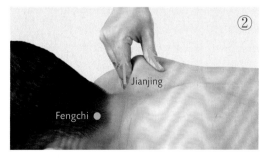

for 1 to 2 minutes each.

❷ Grasping method: Have the patient lying in a prone position. Grasp the Jianjing and Fengchi acupoints.

Additional Steps for Vomiting Caused by Food Stagnation

❶ Kneading method: Knead the Neiguan acupoint using the thumb pulp with slightly more force until soreness is generated.

❷ Circular rubbing method: Have the patient lying in a supine position. Stand on one side of the patient and apply circular rubbing with the palm on the abdomen for 3 to 5 minutes until a warm feeling is generated.

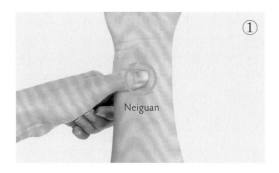

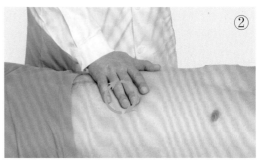

Additional Steps for Vomiting with Liver *Qi* Invading Stomach

❶ Kneading method: Have the patient lying in a prone position. Knead with the thumb pulp on both sides of the Ganshu and Danshu acupoints with slightly more force until the symptoms are relieved.

❷ Pressing-kneading method: Have the patient lying in a supine position. Use the index, middle and ring fingers to press-knead the Zhangmen and Qimen acupoints until soreness is generated.

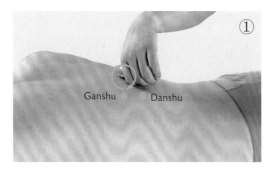

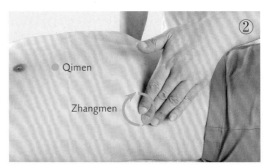

Additional Steps for Vomiting Caused by Spleen and Stomach *Qi* Deficiency

❶ Kneading and to-and-fro rubbing methods: Have the patient lying in a prone position. Knead the Taiyang Bladder Meridian of Foot on the back with the root of the palm, paying attention to the Pishu and Weishu acupoints. Supplement with

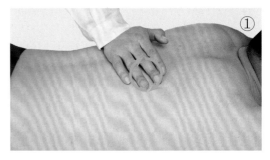

to-and-fro rubbing until the heat generated penetrates through the stomach.

❷ Vibrating method: Have the patient lying in a supine position. Apply the vibrating method with the palm on the Shenque acupoint for 3 to 5 minutes until the heat generated penetrates the back.

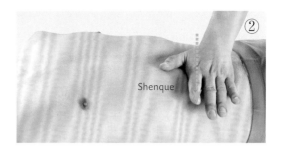

6. Epigastric Pain

Epigastric pain is a pain in the upper abdomen and stomach near the heart fossa. It is often caused by dysfunction of the stomach and the failure of stomach *qi* to descend because of cold pathogen attacking stomach, hurting the stomach due to diet, liver *qi* invading the stomach, and weakness of the spleen and stomach.

Epigastric pain caused by cold pathogen attacking stomach: Sudden onset of stomach pain, disliking cold and preferring warmth, pain decreases when the stomach and abdomen are warmed, pain increases when cold is encountered, no thirst, hot drinks preferred, tongue coating is thin and white.

Epigastric pain caused by liver *qi* invading the stomach: Distension and pain in the stomach and epigastrium, pain extending to the two hypochondrium, pain aggravated when troubled, pain relieved when belching and releasing flatus, chest tightness, long sighing, poor bowel movement, thin white coating on the tongue.

Epigastric pain caused by food stagnation: Pain in the stomach and abdomen, fullness and bloating, belching with fetid odor and acid reflux, or vomiting undigested food, which smells putrid, pain decreases after vomiting, loss of appetite, unpleasant stool, slightly relieved after flatus and passing motions, thick and greasy tongue coating.

Epigastric pain caused by deficiency-cold in spleen and stomach: Dull pain in stomach, vomiting clear water, pain decreases with warmth and pressure, very strong pain in the empty stomach, pain decreases after food intake. Poor appetite, fatigue, or even lack of warmth in the hands and feet, loose stools and white tongue coating.

Basic Steps

❶ Single finger meditation pushing and circular rubbing methods: Have the patient lying in a supine position. Stand on the patient's side and apply the quick and light single finger meditation pushing method on the Conception Vessel on the abdomen. The force applied

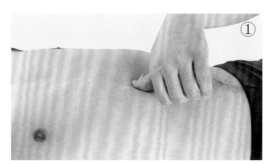

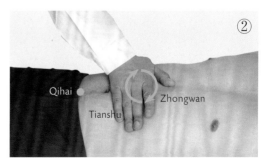

can be slightly harder. Then, apply the circular rubbing method on the abdominal area until the heat generated penetrates the skin.

❷ Kneading method: Apply the kneading method with the palm on the Zhongwan, Tianshu, and Qihai acupoints in a clockwise direction for one minute each.

❸ Single finger meditation pushing method: Have the patient lying in a prone position. Apply the single finger meditation pushing method on both sides of the back spine, along the Taiyang Bladder Meridian of Foot to the Sanjiaoshu acupoint. Repeat this 4 to 5 times.

❹ Pressing-kneading method: Press-knead the Geshu, Pishu, Weishu, and Sanjiaoshu acupoints for 3 to 5 minutes each with more force.

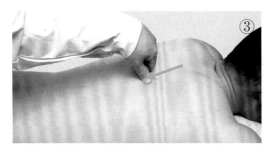
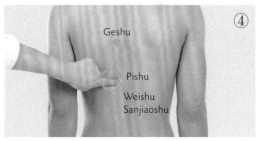

Additional Steps for Epigastric Pain Caused by Cold Pathogen Attacking Stomach

❶ Kneading method: First, locate the pressure point around the patient's Beishu acupoint (usually around the Pishu and Weishu acupoints), then use the pulp of index finger to gently knead the area until the pain disappears or is alleviated.

❷ Finger pressing method: Press the Neiguan acupoint continuously with the thumb pulp with moderate force, until a sore, numb and bloated feeling is generated.

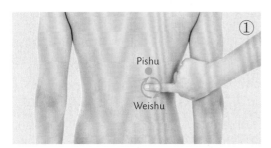
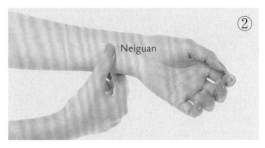

Additional Steps for Epigastric Pain Caused by Liver *Qi* Invading the Stomach

❶ Single finger meditation pushing method: Apply the single finger meditation pushing

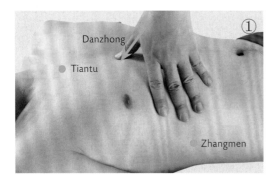
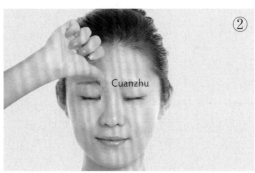

method on the Tiantu, Danzhong, and Zhangmen acupoints for one minute each, ideally until soreness is generated. The speed of pushing should not be too fast.

❷ Pressing method: Press the Baihui, Sishencong, and Cuanzhu acupoints with the thumb pulp in a rhythmic motion for one minute each, until soreness is generated.

Additional Steps for Epigastric Pain Cause by Food Stagnation

❶ Kneading method: Have the patient lying in a prone position. Knead the Danshu acupoint with the thumb pulp for 1 to 2 minutes, ideally to produce soreness.

❷ Pressing method: Press the Shangjuxu and Xiajuxu acupoints with the thumb pulp for 1 to 2 minutes each. The intensity can be slightly higher, ideally to produce a sore, numb and bloated feeling.

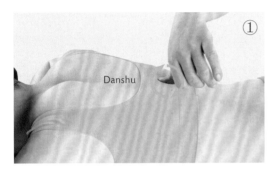
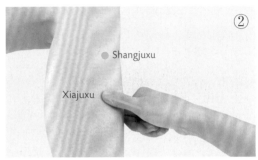

Additional Steps for Epigastric Pain Caused by Deficiency-Cold in Spleen and Stomach

❶ Kneading method: Have the patient lying in a prone position. Knead the Taiyang Bladder Meridian of Foot at the back with the palm, focusing on the Pishu and Weishu acupoints.

❷ Vibrating method: Have the patient lying in a supine position. Apply the vibrating method with the palm on the Shenque acupoint for 3 to 5 minutes, until the heat generated penetrates the skin.

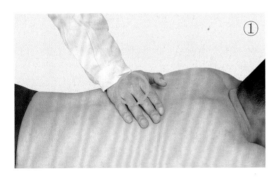
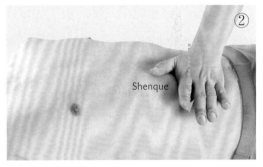

7. Abdominal Pain

Abdominal pain is usually caused by irritation or damage to the intra-abdominal tissue or organs. It can also be a complication from ailments of the chest or systemic diseases. Abdominal pain is a subjective feeling. The nature of the pain and its intensity are not only affected by the severity of the ailment and external stimulation, but also by mental and psychological factors.

Abdominal pain caused by accumulated cold: Acute abdominal pain, aggravated by cold and relieved by heat, decreased diet, no thirst, clear urine, thin white tongue coating.

Abdominal pain caused by deficiency-cold: Continuous abdominal pain that goes on and off, preference for pressure and heat to be applied, condition aggravated by hunger or fatigue, loose stools, being spiritless and shortness of breath, aversion to cold, cold hand and foot, pale tongue with white coating.

Abdominal pain caused by *qi* stagnation: Abdominal distention, constantly shifting pain, pain area extends to the ribs or lower abdomen, condition aggravated by anger, chest tightness, eructation, thin white tongue coating.

Abdominal pain caused by food stagnation: Bloated abdominal pain, hurts when pressed on, nauseous at the sight of food, putrid belching with regurgitation of stomach acid, nausea and vomiting, constipation or diarrhea, greasy tongue coating.

Basic Steps

❶ Pushing method: Have the patient lying in a prone position. Use either a single palm or with both palms stacked to apply force to push the back up and down 3 to 5 times.

❷ Pressing-kneading and palm twisting methods: Have the patient lying in a prone position. Press-knead the Baliao acupoints on both sides of the sacrum with multiple fingers, then apply the palm twisting method on the lumbosacral region for 1 to 3 minutes.

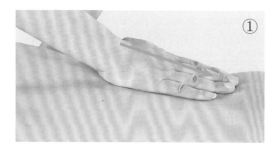
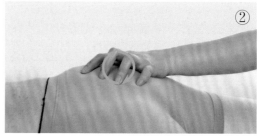

❸ Pushing and kneading methods: Have the patient lying in a supine position. Apply the single palm pushing method from the upper abdomen to the lower abdomen a few times with even force, then stack palms together to knead the abdomen slowly for 4 to 6 minutes. The force applied should be deep but gentle.

❹ Pressing-kneading and circular rubbing methods: Have the patient lying in a supine position. Press-knead in turn along the Conception Vessel, Yangming Stomach Meridian of Foot and Taiyin Spleen Meridian of Foot on the abdomen in a straight line for 3 to 5 minutes. Then, apply the circular rubbing method on the abdomen for 3 to 5 minutes with moderate force, ideally to allow the heat generated to penetrate.

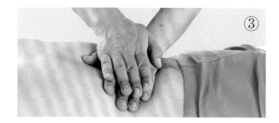
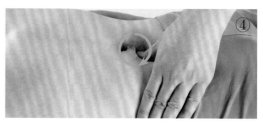

Additional Steps for Abdominal Pain Caused by Accumulated Cold

❶ Pushing method: Have the patient lying in a supine position. Push with the thumb or thenar from the Zhongwan, Xiawan and Qihai acupoints to both sides of the body. Repeat this 7 to 10 times.

❷ Pressing-kneading method: Press-knead the Zusanli, Sanyinjiao, and Taichong acupoints for 1 to 2 minutes each, ideally to generate soreness.

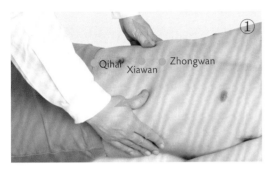

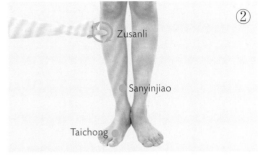

Additional Steps for Abdominal Pain Caused by Deficiency-Cold

❶ Kneading and circular rubbing methods: Use the pulp of the index finger to knead the Daheng and Fujie acupoints for two minutes each. Then apply circular rubbing with the palm in a clockwise direction on the abdomen for two minutes. The intensity of kneading should gradually increase.

❷ Kneading method: Knead the Zusanli acupoint with the thumb pulp for two minutes, ideally to generate soreness.

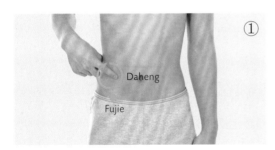

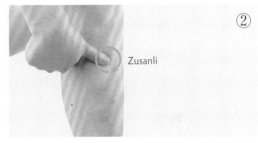

Additional Steps for Abdominal Pain Caused by *Qi* Stagnation

❶ Kneading method: Knead the Zusanli, Sanyinjiao, Taixi, and Taichong acupoints using the thumb pulp, in a clockwise direction. Ideally it should generate soreness.

❷ To-and-fro rubbing method: Use the heel of the palm to rub the foot's Yongquan

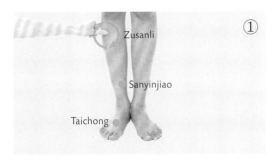

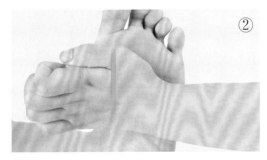

acupoint for two minutes, until the heat generated flows through the lower limbs to the abdomen.

Additional Steps for Abdominal Pain Caused by Food Stagnation

❶ Pressing-kneading method: Have the patient lying in a supine position. Gently press-knead the Liangmen and Tianshu acupoints for two minutes each, until soreness is generated.

  ❷ Kneading method: Use the pulp of thumb or index finger to knead the Fenglong and Xiajuxu acupoints for two minutes each with increasing intensity until soreness is generated.

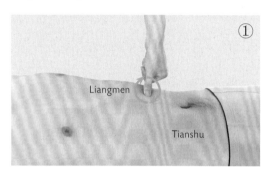
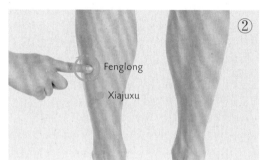

8. Constipation

Constipation refers to prolonged period of no bowel movements, or a short cycle with dry fecal matter, causing difficulty in defecation; or the fecal matter is not hard, but the bowel movement is not smooth. Constipation is caused by diet issues, emotional disorders, old age and weak physique, and invasion of external pathogens. The main cause is usually a dysfunction of the large intestine.

  Constipation caused by heat accumulation in the stomach and intestine: Dry stools and difficulty with defecation, bloating in the abdomen, easily irritable, reddish face with warm body temperature, dry mouth, bad breath, bitter taste in the mouth, limited dark urine, dry tongue with a yellow coating.

  Constipation caused by *qi* stagnation: Dry stools, difficulty with defecation, belly distention, bloated chest and nausea, belching and hiccups, loss of appetite, borborygmus and flatus, tongue coating is thin white or thin yellow, or thin and greasy.

  Constipation caused by deficiency of *yin* and blood: Dry stools, thirst, dysphoria with smothery sensation, weight loss, fatigue, palpitations, dizziness, loss of color in the face, difficulty with defecation, pale tongue with a white coating.

  Constipation caused by *yin* cold congelation and stagnation: Hard and dry stools that are difficult to discharge, pale face, aversion to cold, preference for warmth and pressure, cold abdomen with pain, sore and cold back, clear urine, pale tongue with a white coating.

Basic Steps

❶ Single finger meditation pushing method: Have the patient lying in a supine position. Apply the fast and gentle single finger meditation pushing method on the Zhongwan, Tianshu, and Daheng acupoints for three minutes each, until soreness is generated.

  ❷ Circular rubbing method: Have the patient lying in a supine position. Apply the circular rubbing method with the palm on the abdomen in a clockwise direction for three minutes, ideally to generate a warm feeling.

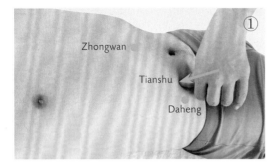
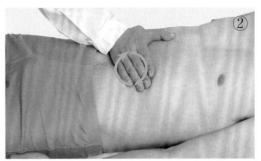

❸ Single finger meditation pushing method: Have the patient lying in a prone position. Apply the fast and gentle single finger meditation pushing method along both sides of the spine from the Ganshu and Pishu to the Baliao acupoints from the top down repeatedly for about three minutes.

❹ Pressing-kneading method: Gently press-knead the Shenshu and Dachangshu acupoints for three minutes each.

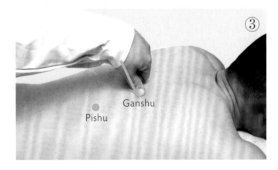
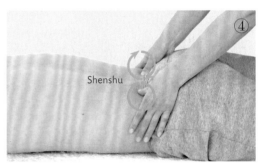

Additional Steps for Constipation Caused by Heat Accumulation in the Stomach and Intestine

❶ Pressing-kneading method: Have the patient lying in a supine position. Press-knead the Shenque acupoint with the heel of the palm for one minute in an anti-clockwise direction until the *qi* is regulated. Then change to clockwise pressing-kneading. This method can cause a borborygmus at the abdomen, inducing flatus and bowel movement.

❷ Pressing-kneading method: Have the patient lying in a prone position. Press-knead

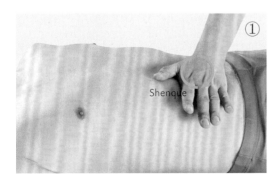
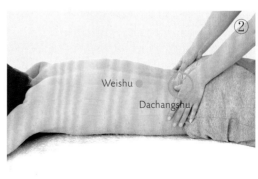

the Weishu, Dachangshu, and Baliao acupoints with the thumb pulp for 3 to 5 minutes with gradual increase in force.

Additional Steps for Constipation Caused by *Qi* Stagnation
❶ Kneading method: Knead the Xingjian and Taichong acupoints for 2 to 3 minutes each, until soreness is generated.
❷ Pressing method: Have the patient lying in a supine position. Stack both hands together to press on the Zhongwan acupoint for 2 to 3 minutes.

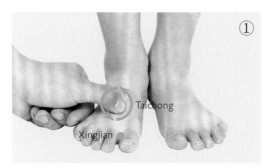
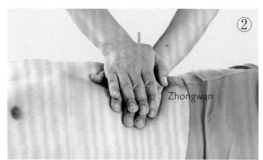

Additional Steps for Constipation Caused by Deficiency of *Yin* and Blood
❶ Pressing-kneading method: Have the patient in either a sitting or supine position. Press-knead the Zusanli acupoint for 2 to 3 minutes with the thumb pulp until soreness is generated.
❷ Pressing-kneading method: Have the patient lying in a prone position. Press-knead the Beishu acupoints (the acupoints on the back where *qi* from the organs are transported, such as Pishu, Xinshu, and Ganshu acupoints) with the thumb for about 2 to 3 minutes each. Then push with the palm from the lumbar to the sacrococcygeal region 5 to 7 times. Pressing-kneading should ideally be executed with more force.

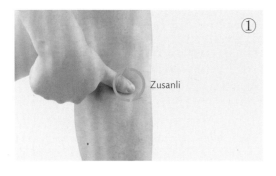
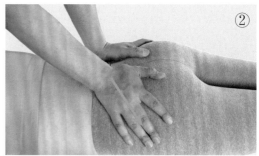

Additional Steps for Constipation Caused by *Yin* Cold Congelation and Stagnation
❶ Pressing method: Have the patient lying in a supine position. Press on the Guanyuan and Qihai acupoints on the abdomen with the palm for two minutes each.

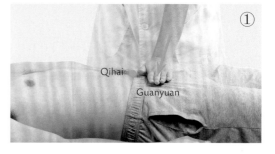

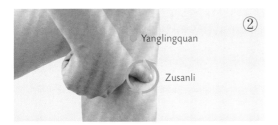

Yanglingquan

Zusanli

② Pressing-kneading method: Have the patient either in a sitting or supine position. Press-knead the Zusanli and Yanglingquan acupoints with the thumb pulp for 2 to 3 minutes each, until soreness is generated.

9. Hiccups

Hiccups are the sound made when gas from the stomach refluxes to the throat. The sound is short, and it is a physiologically common phenomenon caused by the contraction of the diaphragm. Healthy people experience transient hiccups, mainly caused by diet, especially when eating too fast, eating too much, or eating very hot or cold food. Hiccups that occur frequently or continuously for more than 24 hours are known as intractable hiccups. This is commonly seen in certain ailments.

Hiccups caused by reversed flow of *qi* due to stomach cold: Dull and powerful hiccups, chest and gastric discomfort, preference for warmth and the condition is aggravated when exposed to cold, preference for drinking hot beverages, tastelessness in the mouth without thirst, and the tongue coating is white and moist.

Hiccups caused by stagnation of *qi*: Repeated hiccups, often caused by or aggravated by emotional stress, heavy and tight chest, bloated stomach, belching and lack of appetite, borborygmus and flatus, thin and white tongue coating.

Hiccups caused by *yang* deficiency of the spleen and stomach: Low, long, and weak hiccups, shortness of breath, vomiting clear water, abdominal discomfort, preference for warmth and pressure on the affected area, pale face, cold limbs, loss of appetite, fatigues, loose stools, pale tongue with thin white coating.

Hiccups caused by stomach-*yin* deficiency: Short and disjointed hiccups, dry mouth and throat, easily irritated, no appetite, or bloated with little food, dry stool, red tongue with little and dry coating.

Basic Steps

❶ Finger-pressing and kneading and pushing methods: Have the patient lying in a supine position. Finger-press and knead the Quepen acupoint with the middle finger for 3 to 5 minutes until soreness is generated. Then, push the Danzhong acupoint up and down for 3 to 5 minutes.

❷ Circular rubbing method: Have the patient lying in a supine position. Rub the abdomen in a clockwise direction for 3 to 5 minutes, with the Zhongwan acupoint as the focus.

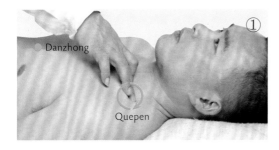

Danzhong

Quepen

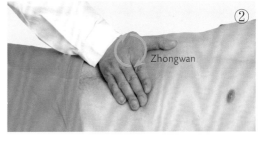

Zhongwan

❸ Single finger meditation pushing and finger-pressing and kneading methods: Apply the single finger meditation pushing method along the Taiyang Bladder Meridian of Foot 3 to 4 times, with emphasis on the Geshu and Weishu acupoints, each pushing for 3 to 5 minutes. Then, focus on finger-pressing and kneading on the Geshu and Weishu acupoints until soreness is generated.

❹ Pushing method: Push with both palms from the sternum outwards in the direction of the ribs, until a warm feeling is generated.

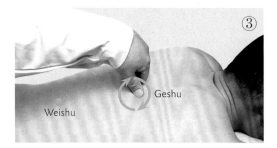

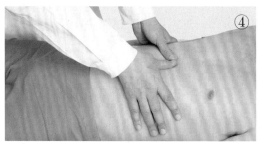

Additional Steps for Hiccups Caused by Reversed Flow of *Qi* Due to Stomach Cold

❶ Pinching method: Have the patient lying in a prone position. Pinch the Governor Vessel and the Taiyang Bladder Meridian of Foot with slightly more force that is comfortable for the patient. Repeat until the hiccups stop or are relieved.

❷ To-and-fro rubbing method: Have the patient lying in a prone position. Rub along the Taiyang Bladder Meridian of Foot to-and-fro with the heel of palms for 3 to 5 minutes, until the heat generated penetrates deeply.

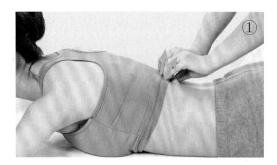

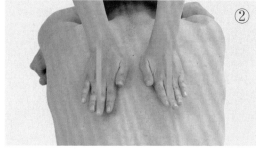

Additional Steps for Hiccups Caused by Stagnation of *Qi*

❶ Pinching method: Have the patient lying in a prone position. Pinch the patient's thoracolumbar spine up and down 3 to 5 times. The force applied can be slightly heavier.

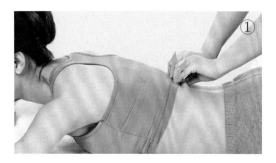

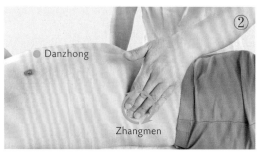

❷ Pressing-kneading and pushing methods: Have the patient lying in a supine position. Use the pulp of index finger, middle finger, and ring finger to gently press-knead the Zhangmen and Danzhong acupoints for 1 to 2 minutes each, until soreness is generated, then apply the pushing method along the ribs on both sides.

Additional Steps for Hiccups Caused by *Yang* Deficiency of the Spleen and Stomach

❶ Single finger meditation pushing method: Have the patient lying in a supine position. Apply the single finger meditation pushing method on the Tianshu acupoint for 2 to 3 minutes. More force can be applied with this method.

❷ Pressing-kneading method: Press-knead the Zusanli acupoint for 2 to 3 minutes with the thumb pulp, until soreness is generated.

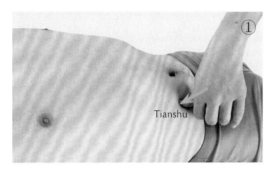
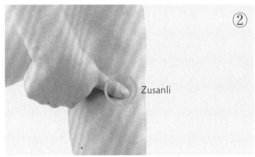

Additional Steps for Hiccups Caused by Stomach-*Yin* Deficiency

❶ Single finger meditation pushing method: Have the patient lying in a supine position. Apply single finger meditation pushing from the top down, starting from the Zhongwan acupoint to the Tianshu and Guanyuan acupoints for three minutes each, ideally to produce soreness.

❷ Pressing-kneading method: Use the thumb pulp to press-knead Zusanli, Fenglong, and Sanyinjiao acupoints with moderate force, ideally to generate soreness.

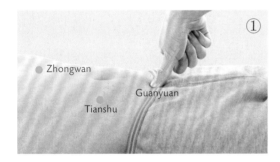
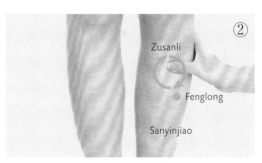

10. Heart Palpitations

Heart palpitations include fright palpitations and severe palpitations, which refer to the patient's feeling of palpitations and disturbances in the heart and can prevent the patient from thinking clearly. It usually manifests itself in the form of paroxysmal, acting up due to emotional fluctuations or fatigue. It often comes with insomnia, forgetfulness, dizziness, tinnitus and other disorders.

Palpitations caused by heart blood deficiency: Palpitations, restlessness, chest tightness, shortness of breath; condition is aggravated when the patient moves; pale face, cold limbs, pale tongue with a white coating.

Palpitations caused by hyperactivity of fire due to *yin* deficiency: Palpitations, restless and easily irritated, insomnia, dizziness, sore and weak knees, feverishness in palms and soles, red tongue with little or no coating.

Palpitations caused by devitalization of heart *yang*: Palpitations, restlessness, chest tightness, shortness of breath; condition is aggravated when the patient moves; pale face, cold limbs, pale tongue with white coating. Usually caused by a long and serious illness that results in the weakening of *yang qi*. The heart cannot be nourished, causing palpitations.

Palpitations caused by stagnant blockade of heart blood: Palpitations, restlessness, tightness and discomfort of the chest, purplish-blue color of nails when heart pains, dark purple tongue or tongue with patches of bruise.

Basic Steps

❶ Single finger meditation pushing method: Have the patient seated upright. Stand on one on side and apply the single finger meditation pushing method on the Yintang acupoint from bottom up and on superciliary arch for 5 to 10 times, ideally to generate a warm feeling.

❷ Pushing and pressing-kneading methods: Push the patient's Qiaogong acupoints with the thumb from top down, the left side first, then the right side, for 2 to 3 minutes each side. Then press-knead the Baihui and Fengchi acupoints for 2 to 3 minutes each.

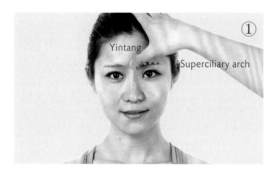
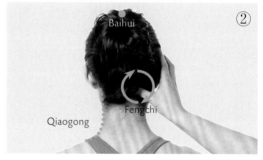

❸ Single finger meditation pushing method: Have the patient lying in a prone position. Apply the single finger meditation pushing method on the Xinshu, Geshu, Ganshu, and Danshu acupoints for 2 to 3 minutes each, until soreness is generated.

❹ Pressing-kneading and circular rubbing methods: Press-knead the Danzhong acupoint with the index finger, then apply the circular rubbing method on the Zhongfu and Yunmen acupoints with the palm for 2 to 3 minutes each. This *tui na* massage should be gentle.

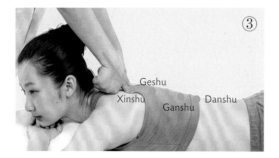
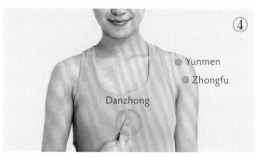

Additional Steps for Palpitations Caused by Heart Blood Deficiency

❶ Kneading method: Have the patient lying in a prone position. Knead the Taiyang Bladder Meridian of Foot with the heel of the palm with slightly more force, focusing on the Xinshu and Geshu acupoints, until a warm feeling is generated.

    ❷ Pressing-kneading method: Press-knead the Xuehai, Zusanli, and Sanyinjiao acupoints with the thumb pulp in a clockwise direction for 2 to 3 minutes, ideally until soreness is generated.

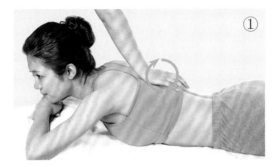
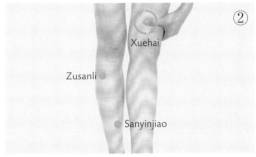

Additional Steps for Palpitations Caused by Hyperactivity of Fire Due to *Yin* Deficiency

❶ Pressing-kneading and to-and-fro rubbing methods: Have the patient lying in a prone position. Press-knead the Shenshu, Xuanshu, and Mingmen acupoints with the thumb pulp, with slightly heavier force until soreness is generated. Then, apply the to-and-fro rubbing method from the Xuanshu acupoint to the Mingmen acupoint, and rub the Baliao acupoints horizontally until the heat generated penetrates the skin.

    ❷ Pressing and palm twisting methods: Press the Sanyinjiao and Taixi acupoints with the thumb pulp for 1 to 2 minutes each, then apply the palm twisting method on the Yongquan acupoint until the sole is warm.

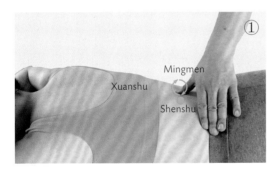
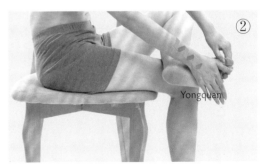

Additional Steps for Palpitations Caused by Devitalization of Heart *Yang*

❶ Pressing-kneading method: Press-knead the Shenmen and Neiguan acupoints with the thumb pulp for 1 to 2 minutes each, until a sore, numb, and bloated feeling is generated.

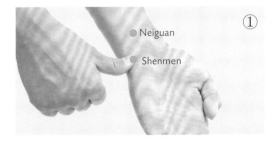

❷ Finger pressing method: Press the Qihu and Wuyi acupoints with the thumb pulp 5 to 10 times each, until a sore, numb, and bloated feeling is generated.

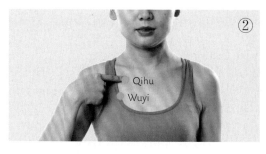

Additional Steps for Palpitations Caused by Stagnant Blockade of Heart Blood

❶ Pressing-kneading method: Have the patient either in a seated or prone position. Press-knead the Jueyinshu and Gaohuang acupoints with the thumb pulp in a clockwise direction for 1 to 2 minutes each, until soreness is generated.

❷ Pinching and finger pressing methods: Have the patient seated in an upright position with the body relaxed. First apply the pinching method on the neck and shoulder muscles, then finger press on the Jianjing, Quepen, and Bingfeng acupoints for 1 to 2 minutes each, until soreness is generated.

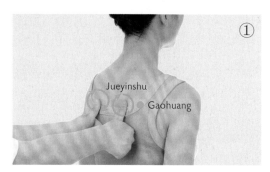

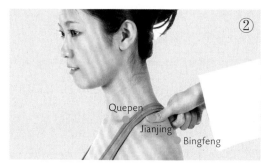

11. Vertigo

Vertigo is a condition in which the patient feels dizzy and is unable to sit or stand, and is often accompanied by other symptoms such as nausea, vomiting and sweating. Those with milder vertigo will feel better after closing their eyes for a while; those who are more severe will feel as if they are on a bumpy ride, with dizziness, inability to stand, and even fainting.

Vertigo caused by hyperactivity of liver *yang*: Dizziness and tinnitus, headache, stiff neck, aggravated when stressed or angered, easily irritated, insomnia or lots of dreams in sleep, reddish face and bitter taste in mouth, red tongue with yellow coating.

Vertigo caused by blood and *qi* deficiency: Vertigo intensifies when in motion or fatigued, pale face, dull lips and fingernails, no shine to the hair, less sleep, being lethargic and withdrawn, poor appetite, pale tongue.

Vertigo caused by liver and kidney-*yin* deficiency: Dizziness, tinnitus and deafness, insomnia, forgetfulness, sore and weak back and knees, lethargy, dysphoria with feverish sensation in chest, palms and soles, reddish tongue, sometimes the body and limbs are cold, pale tongue.

Vertigo caused by phlegm-turbidity obstructing middle-*jiao*: Dizziness, cloudy head, stiff neck, sleeping more but eating less, lethargy and fatigue, chest tightness, nausea, blurred vision, pale tongue with greasy white coating.

Basic Steps

❶ Finger-pressing and kneading and pushing methods: Have the patient either seated or lying in a supine position. Finger-press and knead the Jingming, Cuanzhu, Taiyang, Yuyao, and Sibai acupoints for 1 to 2 minutes each. Then push from the Yintang acupoint to the hairline, before pushing the forehead and orbital area and kneading from the Taiyang acupoint to temporal 5 to 8 times.

❷ Grasping-kneading and finger pressing methods: Use the thumb and the four fingers to grasp-knead both sides of the Fengchi acupoints with relative force, then use the pulp of index finger to press the Fengfu acupoint for 1 to 2 minutes.

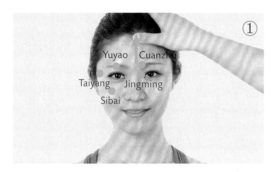
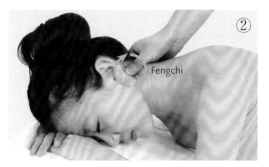

❸ To-and-fro rubbing and pushing methods: Have the patient lying in a prone position. Apply to-and-fro rubbing horizontally on the back with the palm until heat generated penetrates the skin, then push the Taiyang Bladder Meridian of Foot on the back 5 to 10 times.

❹ Pinching method: Have the patient lying in a prone position. Pinch and lift the lower limbs with the thumb and other four fingers for 3 to 5 minutes.

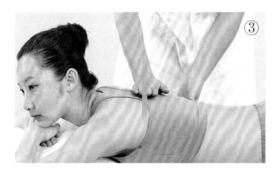
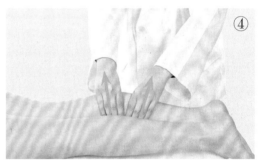

Additional Steps for Vertigo Caused by Hyperactivity of Liver *Yang*

❶ Pinching method: Have the patient lying in a prone position. Pinch the back and lift the

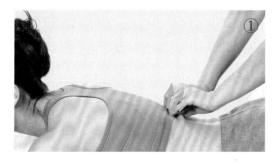
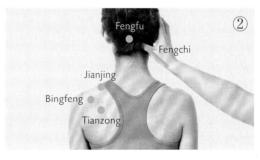

skin upwards, from the lower back upwards. Repeat three times. The force applied should be moderate for the patient to withstand.

❷ Pressing and grasping methods: Press the acupoints in the following order for 1 to 2 minutes each: Fengchi, Fengfu, Jianjing, Tianzong, and Bingfeng. Next, apply the grasping method on the neck and shoulders with increasing force.

Additional Steps for Vertigo Caused by Blood and *Qi* Deficiency

❶ Finger pressing and plucking methods: Have the patient lying in a supine position. Press on the Tianshu and Guanyuan acupoints, and pluck the Quepen and Qihu acupoints for one minute each, until soreness is generated.

❷ Finger pressing method: Have the patient either seated in an upright position or standing. Press on the Xuehai, Liangqiu, and Zusanli acupoints for one minute each, until soreness is generated.

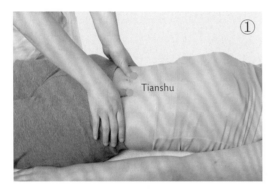
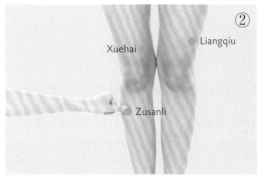

Additional Steps for Vertigo Caused by Liver and Kidney-*Yin* Deficiency

❶ Rolling and kneading methods: Have the patient relax their shoulders. Apply rolling and finger kneading methods interchangeably on the neck and shoulder, placing emphasis on the Jianjing acupoint. Knead until soreness is generated.

❷ Pressing method: Press on the Yongquan acupoint with the thumb pulp for one minute until soreness is generated.

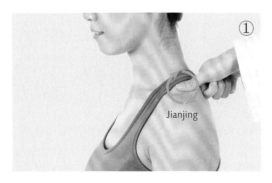
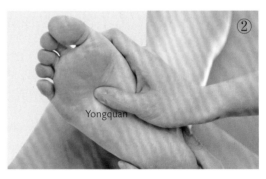

Additional Steps for Vertigo Caused by Phlegm-Turbidity Obstructing Middle-*Jiao*

❶ Grasping and pushing methods: Have the patient standing. Apply the grasping method on the head where the hair is, and apply marginally more strength. Supplement with the pushing method on the Qiaogong acupoints. Push one side before working on the other.

❷ Pressing method: Have the patient either standing or seated. Press the acupoints in the following order for one minute each, until soreness is generated: Xuehai, Zusanli, Yinlingquan, Fenglong, and Gongsun acupoints.

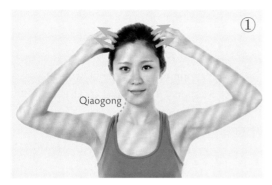

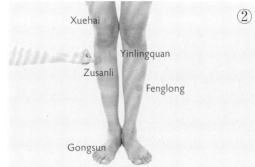

12. Headache

Headache is a common symptom, and may appear alone or in conjunction with other acute and chronic illnesses. There are a variety of reasons for headaches to occur. Traditional Chinese medicine divides them into exogenous type and internal type. Exogenous type are then divided into wind-cold and wind-heat types, while internal type are divided into phlegm-turbidity and blood deficiency types.

Wind-cold type headache: Usually occurs after exposure to cold wind; sometimes the pain stretches to the neck; aversion to wind and cold; the patient likes to have their head wrapped; no thirst, thin white tongue coating.

Wind-heat type headache: Throbbing headache, as though the skull is cracking; aversion to wind and fever, red face and bloodshot eyes, thirst, inflamed throat, dark urine or constipation, thin and yellow coating or a reddish tip of tongue.

Phlegm-turbidity type headache: Throbbing headache, chest distention, fatigue and lack of appetite, increased saliva, nausea, greasy white tongue coating.

Blood deficiency type headache: Headache and dizziness, fatigue, pale face, palpitations, shortness of breath, pale tongue.

Basic Steps

❶ Pressing-kneading and single finger meditation pushing methods: Have the patient seated upright. Use either pressing-kneading method or single finger meditation pushing to massage

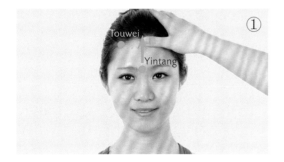

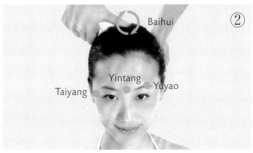

from the Yintang acupoint up towards the hairline and to the Touwei acupoint. Repeat this motion 3 to 4 times.

❷ Pressing-kneading method: Have the patient seated upright. Press-knead the Yintang, Yuyao, Taiyang, and Baihui acupoints for 1 to 2 minutes each, until soreness is generated.

❸ Pinching and grasping methods: Have the patient seated upright. Stand on one side and apply the pinching and grasping methods on the Fengchi and Jianjing acupoints for 2 to 3 minutes each.

❹ Single finger meditation pushing method: Have the patient seated upright. Apply the single finger meditation pushing method along the Taiyang Bladder Meridian of Foot on both sides of the neck from the top in a downward direction for 2 to 3 minutes. The force applied can be slightly heavier.

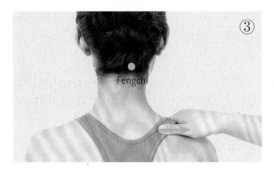
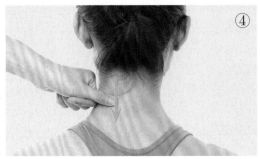

Additional Steps for Wind-Cold Type Headache

❶ Finger-pressing and kneading method: Have the patient seated upright. Stand behind the patient to finger-press and knead the Tianzhu acupoint for 1 to 2 minutes, until soreness is generated.

❷ Finger-pressing and kneading method: Have the patient seated upright. Press and knead the Feishu and Fengmen acupoints with the thumb pulp in a clockwise direction for 1 to 2 minutes each, until soreness is generated.

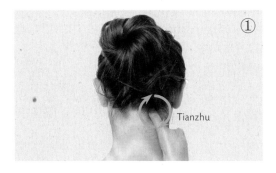
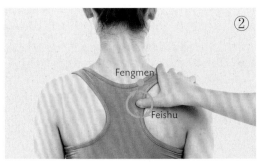

Additional Steps for Wind-Heat Type Headache

❶ Pressing-kneading method: Press-knead the Quchi and Shousanli acupoints with the pulp of index finger for one minute each with slightly more force, ideally to generate soreness.

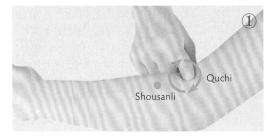

❷ Pressing-kneading and patting methods: Use the thumb pulp to press-knead the Dazhui and Feishu acupoints for one minute each, then apply the patting method on both sides of the Taiyang Bladder Meridian of Foot at the back, until the skin is slightly reddish.

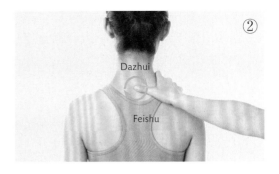

Additional Steps for Phlegm-Turbidity Type Headache

❶ Pressing-kneading and to-and-fro rubbing methods: Use the thumb pulp to press-knead the Pishu, Weishu, and Dachangshu acupoints for three minutes each. Then apply the to-and-fro rubbing method horizontally across the back, straightly rubbing the Governor Vessel until the heat generated penetrates the skin.

❷ Pressing-kneading and circular rubbing methods: Have the patient lying in a supine position. Stands beside the patient and apply the pressing-kneading method with the thumb pulp on the Zhongwan and Tianshu acupoints in a clockwise direction for three minutes each; then apply the circular rubbing method on the abdomen in a clockwise direction for 3 to 5 minutes.

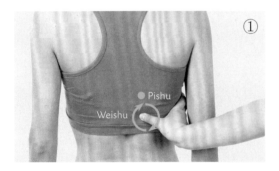
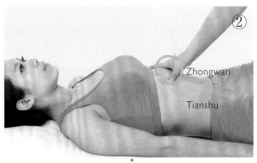

Additional Steps for Blood Deficiency Type Headache

❶ Pressing-kneading and to-and-fro rubbing methods: Have the patient sitting upright. Use the thumb pulp to press-knead the Xinshu and Geshu acupoints for 3 to 5 minutes each. Then apply the to-and-fro rubbing method vertically on the upper back and along the Governor Vessel, until the heat generated penetrates the skin. The force applied should gradually increase.

❷ Circular rubbing method: Have the patient lying in a supine position. Stand on one side and apply the circular rubbing method on the abdomen in a clockwise direction for 3 to 5 minutes.

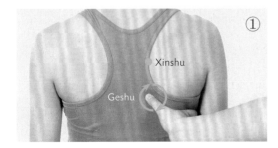
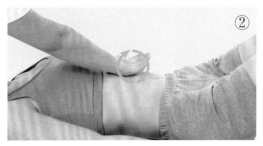

13. Insomnia

Insomnia is a condition where the patient is unable to sleep normally. It is usually characterized by short and light sleep. Patients with minor insomnia find it difficult to fall asleep or experience light sleep, weaving in and out of consciousness and being unable to sleep again after waking up; sufferers of severe insomnia can be awake the entire night.

Heart and spleen deficiency type insomnia: Multiple dreams and light sleep, palpitations and forgetfulness, fatigue, tastelessness, pale face, pale tongue with thin coating.

Insomnia caused by hyperactivity of fire due to *yin* deficiency: Easily irritated and losing sleep, dizziness, tinnitus, thirst with decreased salivation, dysphoria with feverish sensation in chest, palms and soles, reddish tongue; sometimes experiencing wet dreams, forgetfulness, palpitations, and backaches.

Insomnia caused by liver depression transforming into fire: Insomnia, being easily irritated, no appetite, thirst, red eyes, bitter taste in mouth, dark colored urine, constipation, reddish tongue with yellow coating.

Insomnia caused by phlegm-heat attacking internally: Insomnia, chest tightness, cloudy head, being easily annoyed, bitter taste in mouth, dizziness, greasy yellowish tongue coating.

Basic Steps

❶ Single finger meditation pushing and pressing methods: Have the patient seated in an upright position or lying in a supine position. Apply the single finger meditation pushing method on the Baihui, Shenting, and Shangxing acupoints repeatedly 3 to 5 times. This is followed by pressing the Yintang, Cuanzhu, Yuyao, and Taiyang acupoints.

❷ Grasping method: Grasp the area from the prefrontal hairline to the Fengchi acupoints with five fingers 3 to 5 times. Grasp and lift with slightly more force.

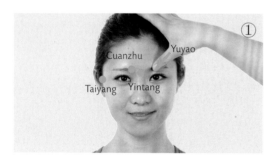
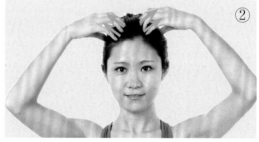

❸ Rolling method: Have the patient lying in a prone position. Apply the rolling method on the back and lumbosacral region with slightly more force, focusing on the Xinshu,

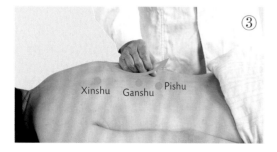
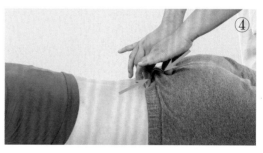

Ganshu, and Pishu acupoints. Roll for about five minutes.

❹ Pinching and pushing methods: Have the patient lying in a prone position. Stand on one side and apply the pinching method on the back in a bottom-up direction 3 to 4 times, then push the Governor Vessel in a top-down direction about 3 to 4 times. Note that the pinching method cannot be performed when the patient is clothed.

Additional Steps for Heart and Spleen Deficiency Type Insomnia

❶ Pressing-kneading method: Use the thumb pulp to press-knead the Shenmen acupoint for 1 to 2 minutes until soreness is generated.

❷ To-and-fro rubbing method: Have the patient lying in a prone position. Stand on one side and apply the horizontal to-and-fro rubbing method on the patient's upper back with the palm. Then, rub along the Governor Vessel vertically until the heat generated penetrates the skin.

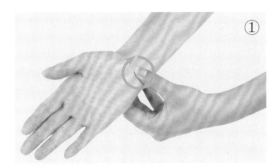
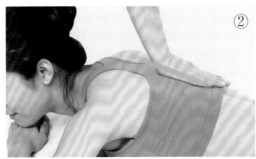

Additional Steps for Insomnia Caused by Hyperactivity of Fire Due to *Yin* Deficiency

❶ Pushing method: Push one side of the Qiaogong acupoint for 1 to 2 minutes with the thumb pulp, then do the same for the other side.

❷ To-and-fro rubbing method: Have the patient lying in a prone position. Stand on one side and apply the horizontal to-and-fro rubbing method on the Shenshu and Mingmen acupoints for 1 to 2 minutes each, until the heat generated penetrates the skin.

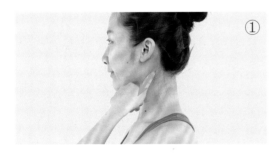
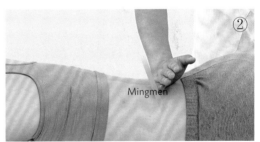

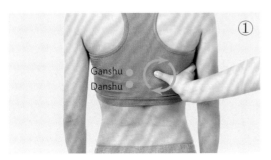

Additional Steps for Insomnia Caused by Liver Depression Transforming into Fire

❶ Pressing-kneading method: Use the thumb pulp to press-knead the acupoints in the following order for 1 to 2 minutes each, ideally generating soreness: Ganshu, Danshu, Qimen, Zhangmen, and Taichong acupoints.

❷ Palm twisting method: Use both hands to apply the palm twisting method on both sides of the ribs for about one minute, until the heat generated penetrates the skin.

Additional Steps for Insomnia Caused by Phlegm-Heat Attacking Internally

❶ Kneading method: Use the index finger and middle finger together to knead the Zhongwan, Tianshu, and Qihai acupoints for one minute each, until soreness is generated. This method can be executed with the thumb pulp too.

❷ To-and-fro rubbing method: Have the patient lying in a prone position. Stand on one side and apply the to-and-fro rubbing method along the Taiyang Bladder Meridian of Foot on the back and the Baliao acupoints on the sacrum, until the heat generated penetrates the skin.

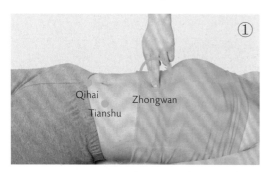
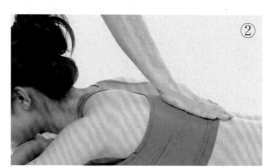

14. Hypertension

Hypertension refers to the increase in systemic circulation arterial blood pressure (systolic and/or diastolic blood pressure) with the systolic blood pressure ≥ 140 mmHg and the diastolic blood pressure ≥ 90 mmHg. It is associated with ailments of the heart, brain, and kidneys, or is a manifestation of organ damage.

Hypertension caused by hyperactivity of liver *yang*: Dizziness, headache, ringing in the ears, reddish face, being easily irritated, cannot sleep soundly at night. Conditions are aggravated when the patient is fatigued or angered, with distending pain in hypochondrium and a bitter taste in mouth. The tongue will also have a yellowish coating.

Hypertension caused by accumulation of turbid phlegm: Dizziness, headache, heavy head, chest tightness, abdominal swelling, vomiting and spitting up sputum, loss of appetite and longer sleeping hours, greasy white tongue coating.

Hypertension caused by hyperactivity of *yang* due to *yin* deficiency: Dizziness, headache, tinnitus, forgetfulness, weak back and knees, hot face and dizziness, dry throat and mouth, a reddish tongue.

Basic Steps

❶ Pushing method: Use either the thumb or both the index and middle fingers to push the Qiaogong acupoint in a downward direction. Start with the left before the right. The duration of a *tui na* massage on each side is about three minutes.

❷ Single finger meditation pushing method: Apply the single finger meditation pushing method on the Yintang acupoint upwards to the hairline. Repeat 4 to 5 times. Next, push around the eye socket from the Yintang acupoint to the Jingming acupoint. Alternate both sides and push 3 to 4 times on each side. The duration is about five minutes. Apply this method with moderate force.

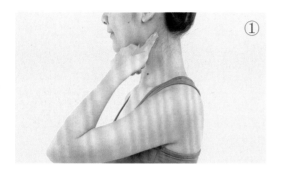

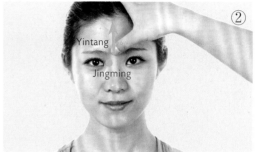

❸ Pressing-kneading method: Apply the pressing-kneading method on the forehead, from the Yintang acupoint to the Taiyang acupoint. Then, apply the pushing method along the Shaoyang Gallbladder Meridian of Foot located at the side of the head. Swipe from the front top to the back bottom for 3 to 5 minutes on each side.

❹ Grasping method: Have the patient seated upright. Apply five-finger grasping method on the head top, and three-finger grasping method on the neck. Continue grasping downwards until the Dazhui acupoint on both sides. Repeat 3 to 4 times. The force applied can be slightly heavier.

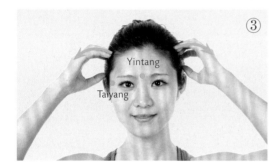

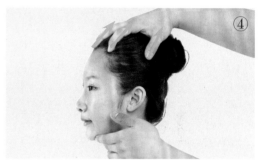

❺ Rolling method: Have the patient lying in a prone position. Apply the rolling method on the patient's Taiyang Bladder Meridian of Foot on the back, focusing on the Jueyinshu, Xinshu, Ganshu, Danshu, and Shenshu acupoints for five minutes.

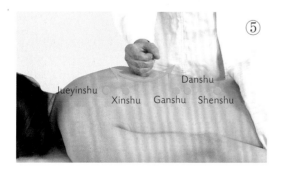

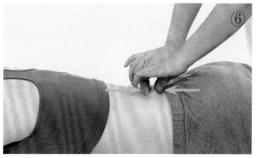

❻ Pinching and pushing methods: Have the patient lying in a prone position. Stand on one side and pinch the back from the bottom upwards. Repeat 3 to 4 times. Then, use palms to push from down upwards along the Governor Vessel on the back. Repeat 3 to 4 times.

Additional Steps for Hypertension Caused by Hyperactivity of Liver *Yang*
❶ Pinching-pressing method: Use the tip of the thumb to nip and press the Taichong and Xingjian acupoints for 2 to 3 minutes each.

❷ To-and-fro rubbing method: Have the patient lying in a prone position. Use the hypothenar to apply the to-and-fro rubbing method on the Ganshu and Shenshu acupoints until the heat generated penetrates the skin.

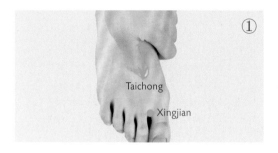
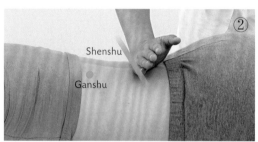

Additional Steps for Hypertension Caused by Accumulation of Turbid Phlegm
❶ Kneading method: Have the patient seated upright. Knead with the thumb pulp on the Fenglong and Jiexi acupoints for 1 to 2 minutes.

❷ Pushing and kneading methods: Push and knead the Zusanli acupoint with the thumb pulp until soreness is generated.

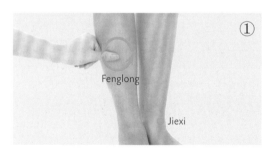
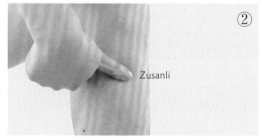

Additional Steps for Hypertension Caused by Hyperactivity of *Yang* Due to *Yin* Deficiency
❶ To-and-fro rubbing method: Have the patient lying in a prone position. Stand on one side

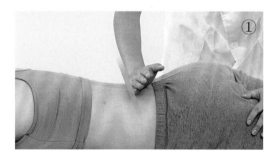
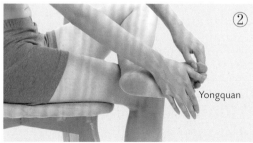

and apply to-and-fro rubbing on the Shenshu and Mingmen acupoints transversely on the back for 1 to 2 minutes.

❷ To-and-fro rubbing method: Adopt a sitting position. Lift one leg up and rest it on the other leg. Then, apply the to-and-fro rubbing method on the Yongquan acupoint with the palm for 1 to 2 minutes, until the heat generated penetrates the skin.

15. Diabetes

Diabetes is a condition characterized by increased food and drink intake, increased diuresis, weight loss, and murky sweet-smelling urine. It occurs due to a *yin* deficiency, an irregular diet, and a failure to regulate emotions and fatigue.

Diabetes caused by fluid consumption due to lung heat: Thirst, an increased water intake, dry mouth and throat, diuresis, reddish sides on the tongue, thin yellow tongue coating.

Diabetes caused by excessive stomach heat: Increased diet with increased frequency of hunger, weight loss, more urine, dry stool, reddish tongue, yellow tongue coating.

Diabetes caused by kidney-*yin* deficiency: Diuresis, more urine, murky urine, fatigue, dizziness and tinnitus, dry mouth and tongue, reddish tongue.

Basic Steps

❶ Rolling method: Have the patient lying in a prone position. Apply a rolling method along the Taiyang Bladder Meridian of Foot on both side of the spine with slightly more force for about six minutes.

❷ Pressing-kneading method: Use the thumb pulp to press-knead the Geshu, Ganshu, Danshu, Pishu, Weishu, Sanjiaoshu, and Shenshu acupoints for 1 to 3 minutes each, until soreness is generated.

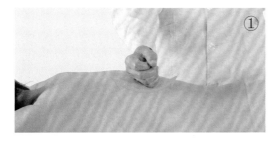
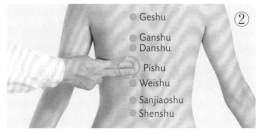

❸ Single finger meditation pushing method: Have the patient lying in a supine position. Apply a single finger meditation pushing method on the Zhongwan, Liangmen, Qihai and Guanyuan acupoints for five minutes with moderate force until soreness is generated.

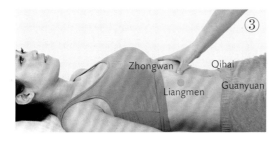
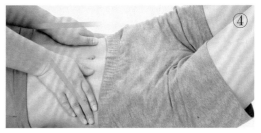

❹ Pushing and to-and-fro rubbing methods: Have the patient lying in a supine position. Push the patient's upper abdomen with the palm for about five minutes, then apply to-and-fro rubbing on the bilateral ribs until the heat generated penetrates the skin.

Additional Steps for Diabetes Caused by Fluid Consumption Due to Lung Heat

❶ Pressing-kneading method: Use the thumb pulp to press-knead the Yangxi and Taiyuan acupoints on the upper limb for 1 to 3 minutes each.

❷ Pressing-kneading method: Use the pulp of index finger to gently press-knead the Lianquan and Chengjiang acupoints for 1 to 3 minutes each.

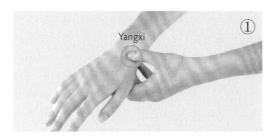
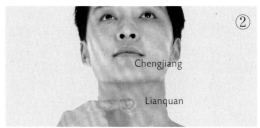

Additional Steps for Diabetes Caused by Excessive Stomach Heat

❶ Pressing-kneading method: Use the thumb pulp to press-knead the Zusanli acupoint with slightly more force for 1 to 3 minutes.

❷ Circular rubbing method: Have the patient lying in a supine position. Stack both hands and apply a circular rubbing method on the abdomen in a clockwise direction with the Shenque acupoint as the center. The strength and amplitude of the massage should gradually increase, and the duration is 2 to 3 minutes.

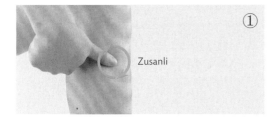
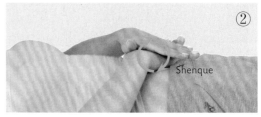

Additional Steps for Diabetes Caused by Kidney-*Yin* Deficiency

❶ Kneading method: Have the patient lying in a supine position. Knead the Qihai, Guanyuan and Zhongji acupoints found along the Conception Vessel with the thumb pulp for 1 to 2 minutes each, until a warm feeling is generated.

❷ Kneading method: Have the patient lying in a prone position. Knead the lumbosacral region with the heel of the palm for about three minutes.

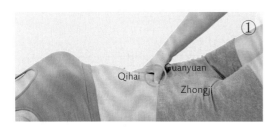
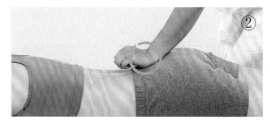

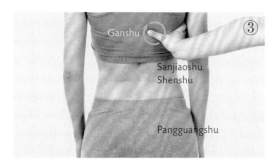
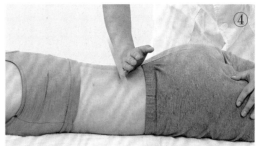

❸ Pressing-kneading method: Use the thumb pulp to press-knead the Ganshu, Sanjiaoshu, Shenshu and Pangguangshu acupoints for 1 to 2 minutes each, until soreness is generated.

❹ To-and-fro rubbing method: Have the patient lying in a prone position. Stand on one side and apply to-and-fro rubbing on the patient's Mingmen, Baliao, and Yaoshu acupoints for 1 to 2 minutes each, until the heat generated penetrates the skin.

16. Coronary Heart Disease

Coronary heart disease is a heart disease caused by coronary artery atherosclerosis that blocks the vascular cavity and leads to myocardial ischemia and hypoxia, and together with functional changes in the coronary arteries, it is collectively called coronary heart disease, also known as ischemic heart disease.

Coronary heart disease caused by *yin* cold congelation and stagnation: An excruciating pain in the chest, heart pain stretching through to the back or back pain stretching through to the heart, cold limbs, pale face, cold sweat in severe case; palpitations and shortness of breath, usually triggered or aggravated by sudden drop in temperature; thin white tongue coating.

Coronary heart disease caused by *qi* stagnation and blood stasis: Chest tightness, periodic dull pain, pain in a locatable spot; condition can be aggravated by negative feelings, usually accompanied by a bloated chest and chest pain; frequent sighing, and a purplish tongue with ecchymosis.

Coronary heart disease caused by phlegm-heat disturbing heart: Shortness of breath, palpitations, fatigue, spontaneous sweating, a bitter taste in mouth, upset feeling, heavy head, dizziness, reddish tongue with a greasy yellow coating.

Coronary heart disease caused by *yang qi* exhaustion: Dull pain in heart or chest tightness, shortness of breath, dizziness, palpitations, fatigue, laziness to speak, aversion to cold, cold limbs, pale face, sweating easily, pale fat tongue with teeth marks on the edge.

Basic Steps

❶ Single finger meditation pushing and to-and-fro rubbing methods: Have the patient lying in a supine position. Apply the single finger meditation pushing method on the Danzhong acupoint with slightly more force until soreness is generated. Then, apply to-and-fro rubbing method on the chest until the heat generated penetrates the skin.

❷ Grasping-kneading method: Used the thumb and the index finger, middle finger, or the other four fingers to grasp-knead the inner muscles of the upper limbs with moderate force for about three minutes.

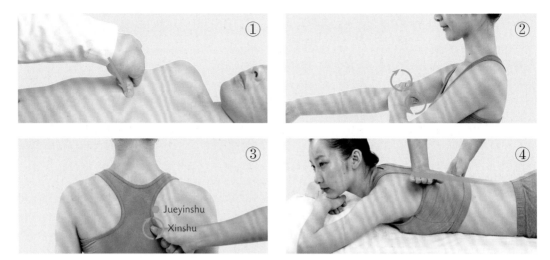

❸ Pressing-kneading method: Press-knead the Xinshu and Jueyinshu acupoints with slightly more force for three minutes each.

❹ To-and-fro rubbing method: Have the patient lying in a prone position. Stand on one side and rub the patient's back to-and-fro with the palm heel until heat generated penetrates the skin.

Additional Steps for Coronary Heart Disease Caused by *Yin* Cold Congelation and Stagnation

❶ To-and-fro rubbing, kneading and pressing-kneading methods: Use the palm heel or the hypothenar to rub and knead the chest 50 times, focusing on the Danzhong and Guanyuan acupoints. Press and knead these acupoints for three minutes until the chest feels warm and the pain is alleviated.

❷ Pressing-kneading method: Have the patient lying in a prone position. Stand on one side and apply the pressing-kneading method on the Zhiyang acupoint with slightly more force for three minutes, until soreness is generated.

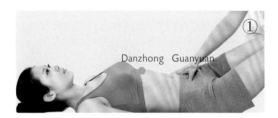
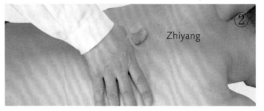

Additional Steps for Coronary Heart Disease Caused by *Qi* Stagnation and Blood Stasis

❶ Pushing method: Use the thumb pulp to push along the patient's Taiyang Bladder Meridian of Foot, from the Feishu acupoint to the Geshu acupoint.

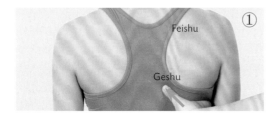
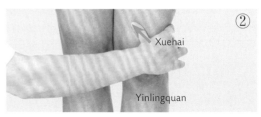

❷ Pressing method: Use the thumb pulp to press on the Xuehai and Yinlingquan acupoints for one minute each, until soreness is generated.

Additional Steps for Coronary Heart Disease Caused by Phlegm-Heat Disturbing Heart
❶ Finger pressing method: Use the thumb pulp to press on the Fenglong acupoint with slightly more force for one minute, until soreness is generated.

❷ Patting method: Pat the back with arched palm for one minute with moderate force.

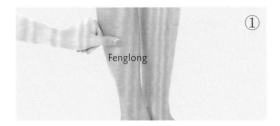

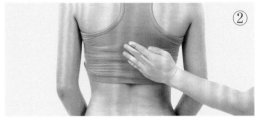

Additional Steps for Coronary Heart Disease Caused by *Yang Qi* Exhaustion
❶ Finger pressing method: Have the patient lying in a supine position. Press the Qihai acupoint for three minutes with slightly more force, until soreness is generated.

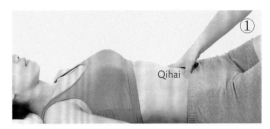

17. Stroke Sequelae

After an acute cerebrovascular attack (stroke), the patient is left half paralyzed and numb, with a drooping eye and mouth, and inaudible speech. This is what is known as stroke sequelae.

Tui na duration: Approximately one minute for each acupoint.

Principles of treatment: To suppress hyperactive liver for calming endogenous wind, relax the tendons, dredge the collaterals, and lubricate the joints.

Points to note: Do not overwork. Have a disciplined routine and balanced diet, and cooperate with the doctor on rehabilitation training.

Steps
❶ Finger-pressing and kneading and grasping-kneading methods: Have the patient lying in

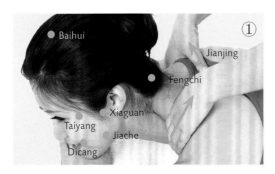

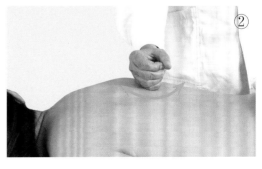

a prone position. Finger-press and knead the Baihui, Taiyang, Xiaguan, Jiache, and Dicang acupoints, then grasp and knead the Fengchi and Jianjing acupoints on both sides of the shoulder.

❷ Rolling method: Have the patient lying in a prone position. Roll along the sides of the spine with slightly more force for about one minute.

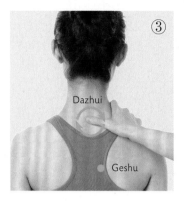
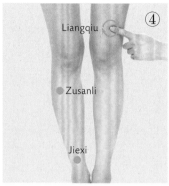
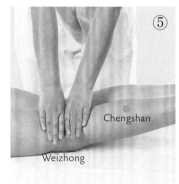

❸ Pressing-kneading method: Use the thumb pulp to press-knead the Dazhui, Geshu, and Shenshu acupoints in a clockwise direction for one minute each, until soreness is generated.

❹ Kneading method: Use the pulp of index finger to knead the Liangqiu, Zusanli, and Jiexi acupoints for one minute each with gradual increase in force, until soreness is generated.

❺ Grasping method: Have the patient lying in a prone position. Grasp the Weizhong, Chengshan, and Kunlun acupoints for one minute each, until a sore, numb, and bloated feeling is generated.

18. Obesity

Traditional Chinese medicine believes that obesity is caused by overeating, functional disorders of the spleen and stomach, and an accumulation of phlegm and dampness. As such, *tui na* massage therapy can help improve the function of the stomach and spleen, eliminates phlegm dampness, and has a good effect on the obesity caused by the functional disorder of the stomach and spleen.

Tui na duration: Approximately one minute for each acupoint.

Principles of treatment: To improve the spleen and stomach in transportation and eliminate dampness and resolve phlegm.

Points to note: Weight loss to a near-normal body weight should be gradual. It should not drop drastically, otherwise the vital *qi* can be damaged and the body's immunity can be compromised.

Steps

❶ Circular rubbing method: Have the patient lying in a supine position. Stand on one side and either use one palm or stack both palms to rub the stomach. Rub in both clockwise and anti-clockwise directions. The area covered should gradually increase before decreasing again. Each direction should be five minutes long.

❷ Grasping method: Have the patient lying in a supine position. Grasp the muscles around the Zhongwan acupoint with one hand and the muscles around the Qihai acupoint with the other. The grasping method covers a large area and should be performed with deep and steady force. Repeat 20 to 30 times.

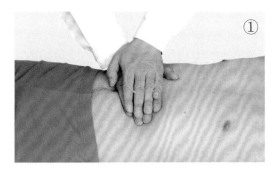
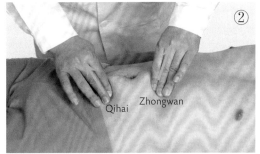

❸ Grasping method: Have the patient seated upright. Stand behind the patient and grasp the muscles around the hypochondrium. Move up and down as you grasp and release. Repeat 20 times.

❹ To-and-fro rubbing and patting methods: Have the patient seated upright. Rub the hypochondrium with the palms forcefully until the heat generated penetrates the skin. Palm-rub the shoulders, back, waist, and lumbosacral region until the heat generated penetrates the skin. Then, apply the patting method with arched palms from top to bottom for 1 to 3 minutes.

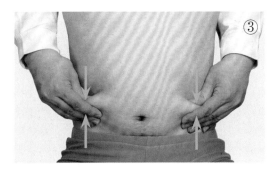
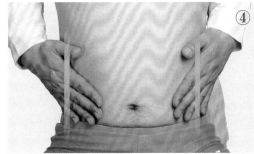

❺ Pinching-grasping method: Have the patient lying in a supine position. Pinch-grasp the patient's limbs with moderate force.

❻ Pressing-kneading and plucking methods: Have the patient either standing or seated upright. Press-knead and pluck the Zusanli and Fenglong acupoints for one minute each, until soreness is generated.

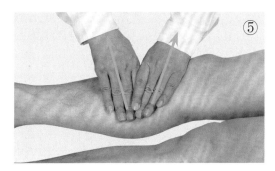
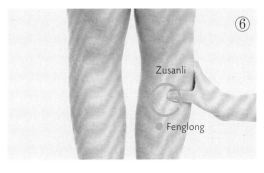

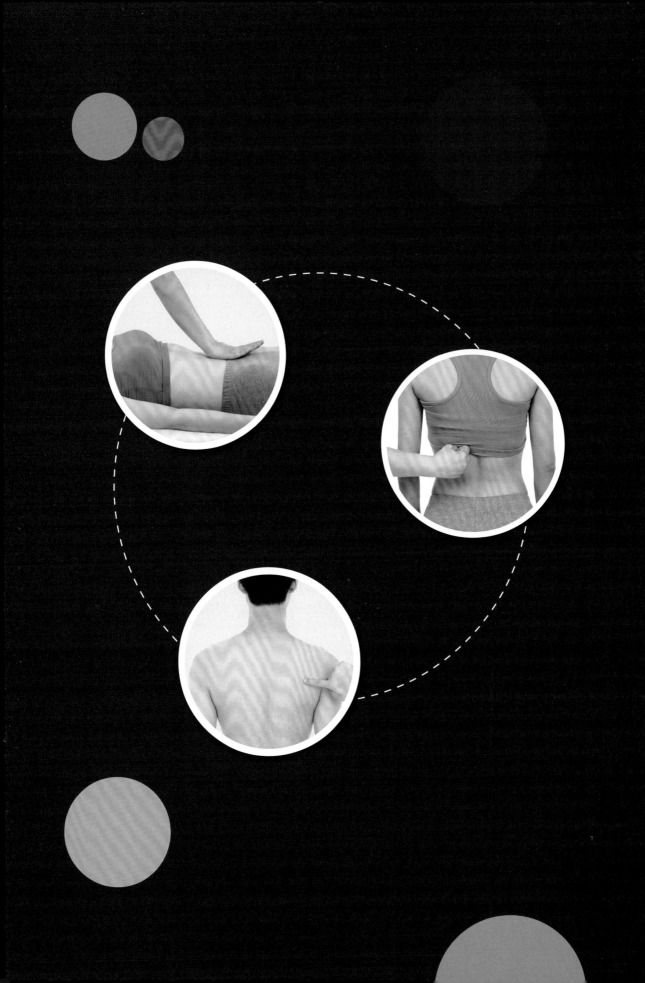

CHAPTER FOUR
Prevention of Male and Gynecological Diseases through *Tui Na*

The fast pace of modern life has put many people in sub-optimal health, including male and gynecological conditions. Due to the taboo that often surrounds such problems, people can be reluctant to go to hospital, which will prolong the condition in the long run, and also affect marital relations. The *tui na* massage techniques introduced in this chapter will help to solve these distressing problems and restore normality.

Note: Some photographs in the book do not have the acupoints marked out due to the angle at which they were taken. Please refer to the appendix for the list of commonly used acupoints in *tui na*. You may wish to follow the step-by-step instructions or use only some of them based on your condition. Massage both acupoints if they are symmetrically distributed on the body.

1. Menstrual Disorders

Menstrual disorders refer to pathological changes in menstruation due to shifts in cycle, quantity, color, and quality, including pre-menstruation, late menstruation, irregular succession, or excessive or too little menstruation.

Blood heat type menstrual disorders: Pre-menstruation, high volume, deep red or purple color, thick texture, irritability, red tongue with yellow coating.

Blood cold type menstrual disorders: Late menstruation, low volume, dark red color, pain in the abdomen, conditions alleviated by heat, cold limbs and an aversion to cold, pale face, light tongue with thin yellow coating.

***Qi* and blood weakness type menstrual disorders:** Empty pain in the abdomen, withered face, dry skin, palpitations and dizziness, light tongue with a thin coating.

***Qi* stagnation type menstrual disorders:** Late menstruation, low volume, normal or dark red color, distension and pain in the abdomen, chest tightness, breast distension and hypochondriac pain, dark red tongue.

Basic Steps

❶ Pressing-kneading method: Have the patient lying in a supine position. Press-knead the Qihai, Guanyuan, and Zhongji acupoints with the thumb pulp for 1 to 3 minutes each. The force applied should gradually increase, until soreness is generated.

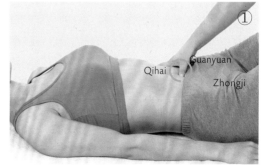

❷ To-and-fro rubbing method: Have the patient lying in a supine position. Apply to-and-fro rubbing on the abdomen in a clockwise direction with the palm for 3 to 5 minutes, until a warm feeling is generated.

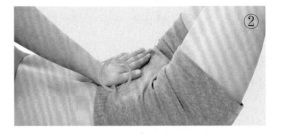

❸ Single finger meditation pushing method: Have the patient lying in a prone position. Apply the single finger meditation pushing method on the Taiyang Bladder Meridian of Foot located along both sides of the spine, placing emphasis on the Pishu, Ganshu, and Shenshu acupoints for 1 to 3 minutes each, until soreness is generated.

❹ Pressing-kneading method: Have the patient seated upright or lying in a supine position. Press-knead the Sanyinjiao, Taichong, and Taixi acupoints for 1 to 3 minutes each, until soreness is generated.

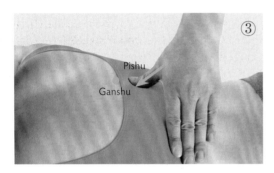

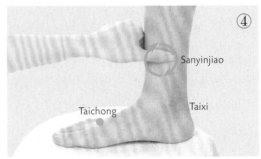

Additional Steps for Blood Heat Type Menstrual Disorders

❶ Pressing-kneading method: Press-knead the Dadun, Xingjian, Yinbai, and Jiexi acupoints with the thumb pulp for 1 to 3 minutes each. The force applied should gradually increase, until soreness is generated.

❷ Pressing-kneading method: Have the patient lying in a prone position. Press-knead the Weishu and Dachangshu acupoints with both palm heels for 1 to 3 minutes each, until soreness is generated.

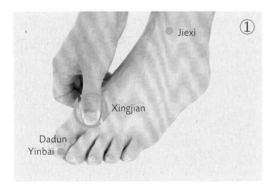

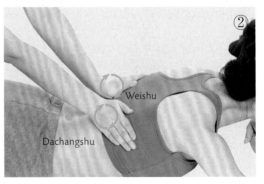

Additional Steps for Blood Cold Type Menstrual Disorders

❶ Pressing method: Have the patient lying in a supine position. Press the Shenque acupoint with the heel of the palm for 3 to 5 minutes until the abdomen feels warm.

❷ To-and-fro rubbing method: Have the patient lying in a supine position. Rub the Governor Vessel on the back and the Shenshu and Mingmen acupoints with the palm heel repeatedly for 3 to 5 minutes each, until the heat generated penetrates the skin.

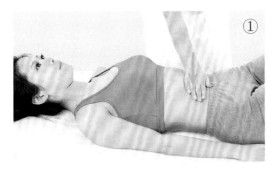 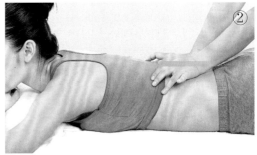

Additional Steps for *Qi* and Blood Weakness Type Menstrual Disorders

❶ Pressing-kneading method: Have the patient standing. Press-knead the Zusanli acupoint with the thumb pulp for 1 to 2 minutes with slightly more force, until soreness is generated.

    ❷ Pressing-kneading method: Have the patient lying in a prone position. Press-knead the Weishu acupoint with the thumb pulp in a circular motion for 1 to 2 minutes.

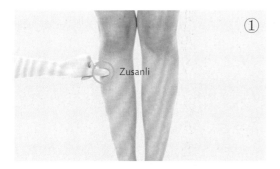 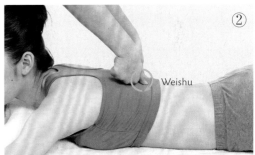

Additional Steps for *Qi* Stagnation Type Menstrual Disorders

❶ Pressing-kneading method: Have the patient lying in a supine position. Press-knead the Zhangmen acupoints with the thumb pulp for 1 to 2 minutes until soreness is generated.

    ❷ Pressing-kneading method: Have the patient seated upright. Press-knead the Geshu acupoint with the thumb pulp for 1 to 2 minutes until soreness is generated. This method can be executed on both sides of the back simultaneously.

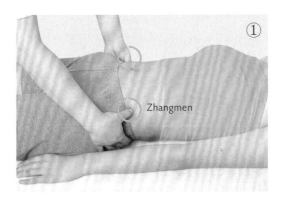 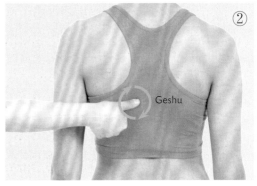

2. Menstrual Pain

This is a condition that occurs before, after, or during the menstruation with pain and swelling in the lower abdomen, accompanied by back pain or other discomfort. Primary dysmenorrhea refers to dysmenorrhea without organic lesions of the reproductive organs; secondary dysmenorrhea refers to dysmenorrhea caused by pelvic conditions such as endometriosis and adenomyosis.

Cold-damp stagnation and congelation type menstrual pain: Cold and pain in the lower abdomen, sometimes causing lumbar pain; condition is alleviated by heat; menstrual discharge is less, dark with blood clots, chills, loose stools.

***Qi* stagnation and blood stasis type menstrual pain:** Premenstrual or menstrual abdominal pain, little menstrual discharge, discharge that is not smooth, dark purple blood with clots; condition is alleviated if the clots are discharged, chest tightness, breast swelling and pain.

Liver and kidney deficiency type menstrual pain: Post-menstrual abdominal pain, light colored blood, little menstrual discharge, lumbar aches, dizziness, tinnitus.

***Qi* and blood deficiency type menstrual pain:** Constant pain in the abdomen during or after menstruation, reduced by pressing; light-colored menstruation, thin menstrual discharge, pale face, fatigue, light tongue with thin coating.

Basic Steps

❶ Circular rubbing method: Have the patient lying in a supine position. Rub the abdomen in a clockwise direction with the palm for about five minutes, until the heat generated penetrates the skin.

❷ Pressing-kneading method: Have the patient lying in a supine position. Press-knead the Qihai, Guanyuan, and Zhongji acupoints with the thumb pulp for 3 to 5 minutes each, until soreness is generated.

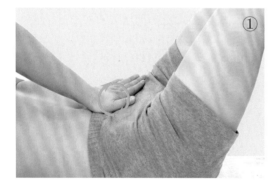

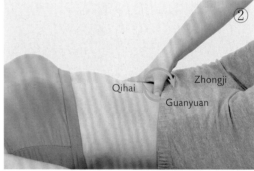

❸ Rolling method: Have the patient lying in a prone position. Apply the rolling method on both sides along the spine and the lumbosacral area. Place your palm closely on the patient when exerting strength. The duration of this massage is about five minutes.

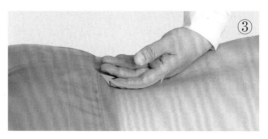

❹ Pressing-kneading and to-and-fro rubbing methods: Have the patient lying in a prone position. Press-knead the Shenshu and Baliao acupoints with the thumb pulp until soreness is generated. The force applied during the pressing-kneading method should gradually increase, until the heat generated penetrates the skin. Then, apply the to-and-fro rubbing method on the lumbosacral area and Baliao acupoints.

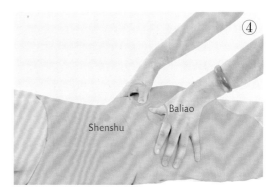

Additional Steps for Cold-Damp Stagnation and Congelation Type Menstrual Pain

❶ To-and-fro rubbing method: Have the patient lying in a prone position. Rub the lumbosacral area vertically, then rub the Shenshu and Mingmen acupoints transversely until the heat generated penetrates the skin. The duration for rubbing for each area is about 3 to 5 minutes.

❷ Pressing-kneading method: Press-knead the Xuehai and Sanjinjiao acupoints for 1 to 3 minutes each, until soreness is generated.

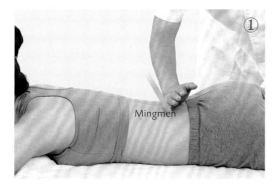

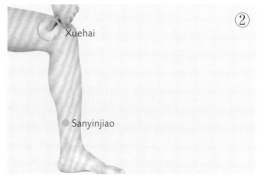

Additional Steps for *Qi* Stagnation and Blood Stasis Type Menstrual Pain

❶ Pressing-kneading method: Have the patient lying in a supine position. Press-knead the Qimen and Zhangmen acupoints with the thumb pulp for 1 to 3 minutes each, until soreness is generated.

❷ Pressing-kneading method: Press-knead the Sanyinjiao acupoint with the thumb pulp for 1 to 3 minutes each. The force applied can be slightly more, until soreness is generated.

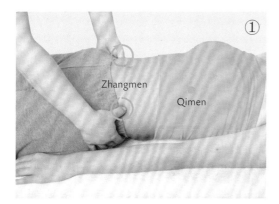

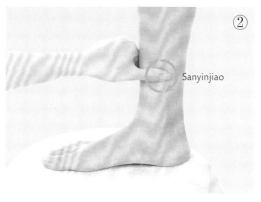

Additional Steps for Liver and Kidney Deficiency Type Menstrual Pain

❶ Pressing-kneading method: Have the patient lying in a prone position. Press-knead the Ganshu acupoint with either the heel of the palm or two palms stacked on top of each other for 1 to 2 minutes, until soreness is generated.

❷ Pressing-kneading method: Have the patient seated upright. Press-knead the Zhaohai, Taixi, and Yongquan acupoints with the thumb pulp for 1 to 2 minutes each, until soreness is generated.

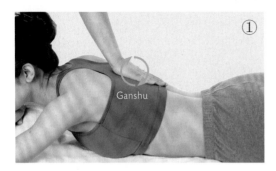
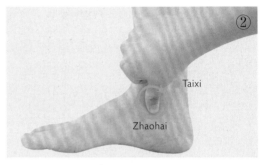

Additional Steps for *Qi* and Blood Deficiency Type Menstrual Pain

❶ Circular rubbing and pressing-kneading methods: Have the patient lying in a supine position. Stand on one side and rub the patient's abdomen in a clockwise direction with the palm. Then, press-knead the Zhongwan acupoint with the thumb for 2 to 3 minutes.

❷ Pressing-kneading method: Have the patient seated upright. Press-knead the Zusanli acupoint with the thumb pulp for 2 to 3 minutes, until soreness is generated.

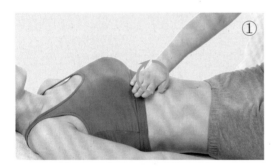
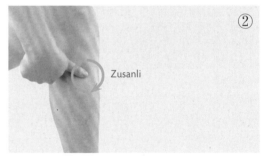

3. Amenorrhea

Amenorrhea refers to the absence of menstruation after the age of 18, or a lack of periods for more than three months (except in the case of pregnancy), in some cases accompanied by symptoms such as dizziness and tinnitus, lumbago, and weakness in limbs.

Liver and kidney deficiency type amenorrhea: The woman has not yet menstruated at the age of 18; late menarche or late menstruation, little discharge with a light color, gradually leading to amenorrhea; weak physique, sore and weak back, dizziness and tinnitus or dry mouth and throat, dysphoria with feverish sensation in chest, palms and soles, periodic sweating and night sweats, dark red cheeks, red tongue or light tongue with little coating.

***Qi* stagnation and blood stasis type amenorrhea:** Menstruation does not occur for several months; feeling depressed, being easily irritated, fullness in the chest, distension and pain in the lower abdomen or pain when massaging the abdomen, purple and dark tongue sides, sometimes with petechia.

***Qi* and blood weakness type amenorrhea:** Menstruation is gradually delayed and eventually stops, with little discharge, accompanied by dizziness, palpitations, shortness of breath, tiredness, loss of appetite, loss of hair shine or easy hair loss, skinny and withered physique, light tongue with little or thin white coating.

Phlegm-dampness stagnation and blockade type amenorrhea: Menstruation stops, weight gain, fullness in the chest, nausea and influx of phlegm, fatigue, white discharge, swollen face and feet, white greasy tongue coating.

Basic Steps

❶ Circular rubbing method: Have the patient lying in a supine position. Apply circular rubbing on their abdomen. Keep the massage deep and slow.

❷ Pressing-kneading method: Press-knead the Xuehai, Zusanli, and Sanyinjiao acupoints in a clockwise direction for two minutes each, until soreness is generated.

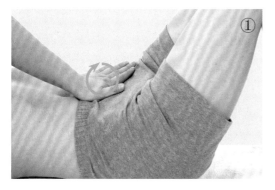
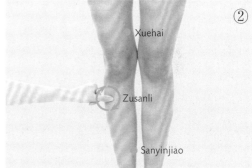

❸ Single finger meditation pushing method: Have the patient lying in a prone position. Apply single finger meditation pushing on both sides of the spine, placing emphasis on the Ganshu, Pishu, and Shenshu acupoints for 1 to 2 minutes each with slightly more force, until soreness is generated.

❹ Rolling method: Have the patient lying in a prone position. Apply the rolling method on both sides of the spine, placing emphasis on the Ganshu, Pishu, and Shenshu acupoints with slightly more force, until soreness is generated.

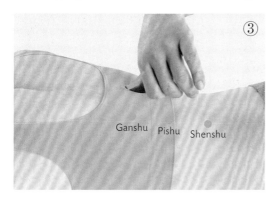
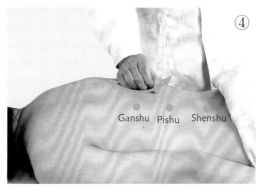

Additional Steps for Liver and Kidney Deficiency Type Amenorrhea

❶ To-and-fro rubbing method: Have the patient lying in a prone position. Apply to-and-fro rubbing with the palm transversely on the Pishu and Weishu acupoints on the back, and Shenshu and Mingmen acupoints in the lumbosacral area, until the heat generated penetrates the skin.

❷ To-and-fro rubbing method: Have the patient lying in a prone position. Rub the Governor Vessel on the back vertically with both palms, then rub the sides of the abdomen until the heat generated penetrates the skin.

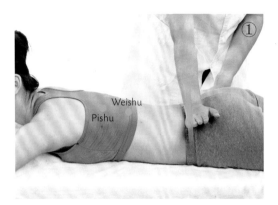
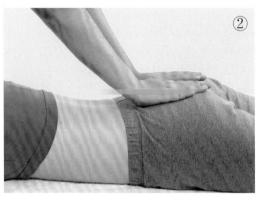

Additional Steps for *Qi* Stagnation and Blood Stasis Type Amenorrhea

❶ Pressing-kneading method: Press-knead both sides of the Zhangmen and Qimen acupoints with pulp of both thumbs for 1 to 3 minutes each, until a sore, numb, and bloated feeling is generated.

❷ Pinching-kneading method: Pinch-knead the Taichong and Xingjian acupoints with the tip of the thumb for 1 to 3 minutes each, until soreness is generated.

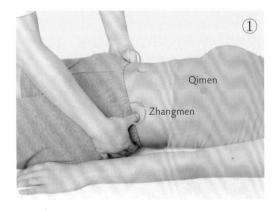
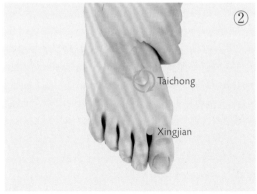

Additional Steps for *Qi* and Blood Weakness Type Amenorrhea

❶ To-and-fro rubbing method: Have the patient lying in a prone position. First, rub the Governor Vessel on the back vertically, then rub the lumbosacral area transversely, until the lower abdomen feels warm.

❷ Pressing-kneading method: Have the patient lying in a prone position. Press-knead the Baliao acupoints with the heel of the palm for 1 to 2 minutes, until the treatment area feels warm.

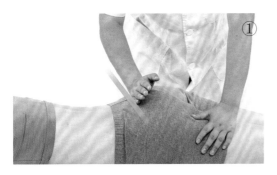

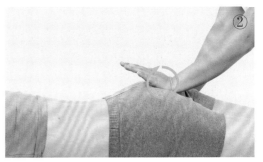

Additional Steps for Phlegm-Dampness Stagnation and Blockade Type Amenorrhea

❶ Pressing-kneading method: Have the patient lying in a prone position. Press-knead the Baliao acupoints with the pulp of both thumbs until soreness is generated.

   ❷ To-and-fro rubbing method: Have the patient lying in a prone position. Rub the back and lumbosacral area transversely until the heat generated penetrates the skin.

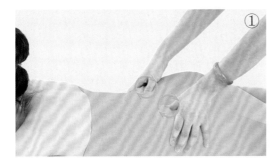

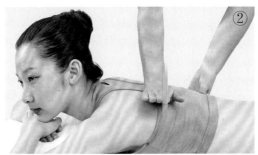

4. Menopausal Syndrome

Menopausal syndrome refers to a series of conditions dominated by severe neurological dysfunction and metabolic disorders caused by diminished ovarian function and decreased estrogen levels in women around the time of menopause. Most of the symptoms can be relieved on their own, but severe cases can affect life and work.

   Tui na **duration:** 2 to 5 minutes for each area.

   Principles of treatment: To regulate *qi* and blood, condition *yin* and *yang*.

   Points to note: Pay attention to psychological treatment for self-strengthening, regulating one's mood and cravings, and being mindful of one's living conditions.

Steps

❶ Single finger meditation pushing, pushing, and pressing-kneading methods: Apply the single finger meditation pushing method on the forehead for five minutes, then push the forehead and face 5 to 10 times, finally press-knead the Taiyang and Baihui acupoints with moderate force for one minute each.

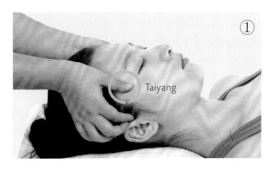

❷ Palm kneading method: Have the patient lying in a supine position. Apply palm kneading on the Danzhong, Qihai, and Guanyuan acupoints for two minutes each with moderate force, until the heat generated penetrates the skin.

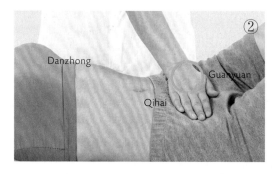

❸ Circular rubbing method: Have the patient lying in a supine position. Rub the upper and lower abdomen in a circular motion for 2 to 5 minutes.

❹ Grasping and grasping-kneading methods: Have the patient seated upright. Apply the grasping method on the patient's head for two minutes, then grasp-knead the neck for two minutes, and finally grasp the Jianjing acupoint 5 to 10 times. The Jianjing acupoint can be massaged simultaneously on both sides.

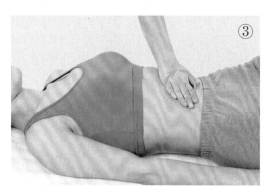
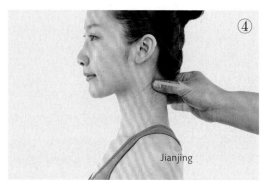

❺ Pressing-kneading method: Press-knead the Jueyinshu, Geshu, Ganshu, Pishu, and Mingmen acupoints with the pulp of the index finger for two minutes each.

❻ To-and-fro rubbing and pushing methods: Push the Governor Vessel and the Taiyang Bladder Meridian of Foot on the back with the heel of the palm, then rub the lumbosacral area and the Shenshu and Mingmen acupoints transversely until the heat generated penetrates the skin.

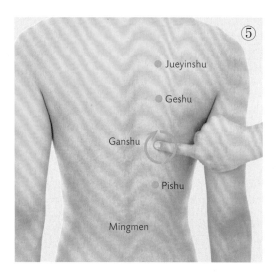
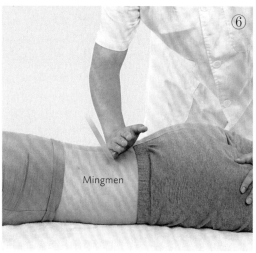

5. Leukorrhea

This is a condition in which the amount of leukorrhea is high, or the color, quality, and odor are abnormal. It is accompanied by the manifestation of systemic or local symptoms. The main cause is acute and chronic inflammation of the reproductive system, such as vaginitis and cervicitis.

Tui na duration: 1 to 2 minutes for each acupoint.

Principles of treatment: To harmonize *yin* and *yang*, nourish the kidneys, and calm the mind.

Points to note: Pay attention to hygiene, and keep the genitals clean.

Steps

❶ Circular rubbing method: Have the patient lying in a supine position. Stand on the side and apply circular rubbing on the abdomen in an anti-clockwise direction. Move around the abdomen in a clockwise direction. Keep the rubbing deep and slow.

❷ Single finger meditation pushing method: Have the patient lying in a supine position. Stand on the side and apply the single finger meditation pushing method on the Zhongwan, Qihai, Guanyuan, and Zhongji acupoints for two minutes each. The force applied should be slow, steady, and even.

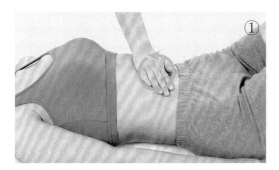
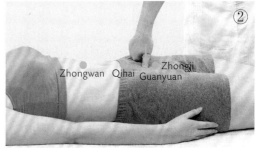

❸ Vibrating method: Have the patient lying in a supine position. Use the palm to apply the vibrating method on the abdomen. Keep the frequency of the vibration slightly fast, and the duration about two minutes long.

❹ Pressing-kneading method: Press-knead the Zhangmen and Qimen acupoints with the thumb pulp for one minute each; press-knead the Daimai acupoints for two minutes. The acupoints on both sides of the body can be massaged simultaneously.

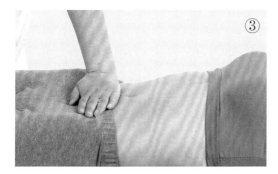
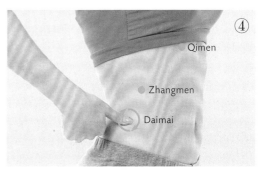

❺ Single finger meditation pushing method: Have the patient lying in a prone position. Apply single finger meditation pushing along the two sides of the spine, focusing on the Ganshu, Pishu, and Shenshu acupoints for 1 to 2 minutes each. Keep the pushing steady.

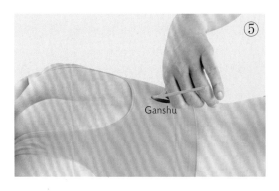

❻ Rolling method: Have the patient lying in a prone position. Apply the rolling method on the lumbosacral area for 1 to 2 minutes, keeping the force deep and even.

❼ Pressing-kneading method: Press-knead the Xuehai, Zusanli, and Sanyinjiao acupoints with the thumb pulp for two minutes each, until soreness is generated.

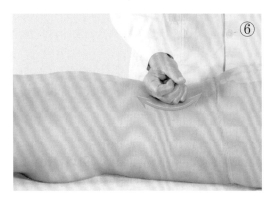

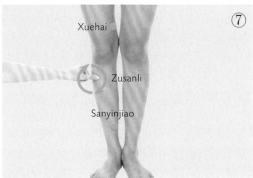

6. Postpartum Hypogalactia

Postpartum hypogalactia is mostly caused by physical weakness and insufficient sources of *qi* and blood generation. *Tui na* massage treatment should focus on regulating and nourishing *qi* and blood, dredging meridians and relieving depression.

Qi and blood weakness type postpartum hypogalactia: Postpartum milk is scarce or even completely absent, milk is thin, breasts are soft, no feeling of fullness; fatigued, and decreased food consumption, pale face, light tongue with little coating.

Liver *qi* stagnation type postpartum hypogalactia: Postpartum milk is astringent and thick, or no lactation; breasts are hard and painful; feeling down and depressed, chest distension, loss of appetite, sometimes slight heat in the body; tongue coloration is normal with thin yellow coating.

Basic Steps

❶ Kneading and circular rubbing methods: Have the patient standing. Place palms on the breasts to knead and rub gently. This includes massaging the Rugen, Tianxi, Shidou, Wuyi, and Danzhong acupoints for 1 to 2 minutes each.

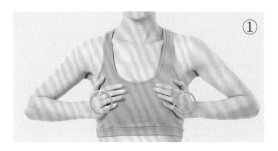

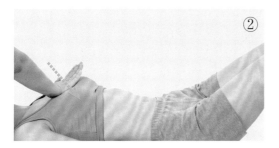
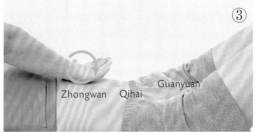

❷ Pressing and vibrating methods: Have the patient lying in a supine position. Press the top and the sides of the breast gently with the palm, focusing the strength on the palm. Then, apply the vibrating method for 1 to 2 minutes.

❸ Pushing and pressing-kneading methods: Use both hands to push from the Xuanji acupoint to the Zhongwan acupoint along the Conception Vessel five times. Then, use the palm to press-knead the Zhongwan, Qihai, and Guanyuan acupoints for three minutes each.

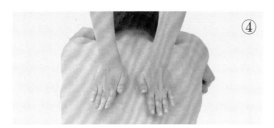

❹ Pushing method: Have the patient lying in a prone position. Use the heel of the palms to push from the Feishu acupoint to the lumbosacral area, along the Taiyang Bladder Meridian of Foot five times. Apply a moderate amount of lubricant for this massage.

Additional Steps for *Qi* and Blood Weakness Type Postpartum Hypogalactia

❶ Single finger meditation pushing and patting methods: Apply the single finger meditation pushing method to push the Ganshu, Pishu, and Weishu acupoints, then apply the patting method along both sides of the Taiyang Bladder Meridian of Foot with a slow speed and even force.

❷ Finger pressing method: Press the Zusanli and Xuehai acupoints with the thumb pulp for 1 to 3 minutes each. Apply slightly more force, until a sore, numb, and bloated feeling is generated.

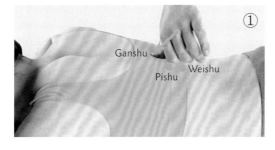
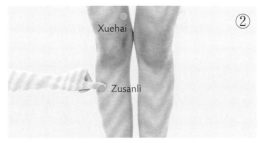

Additional Steps for Liver *Qi* Stagnation Type Postpartum Hypogalactia

❶ Palm twisting method: Place both palms under the armpits and apply the palm twisting method on the ribs 3 to 5 times, until the skin starts to feel warm.

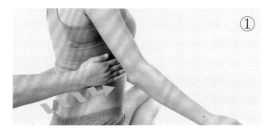

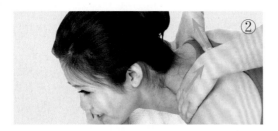

❷ Grasping method: Have the patient lying in a prone position. Grasp and lift the Jianjing acupoints with both hands 3 to 5 times with moderate force.

7. Acute Mastitis

Acute mastitis is an acute purulent infection of the breast, which is an inflammation of the connective tissue in and around the milk ducts. The main symptoms are fever, chills, redness, swelling, heat and pain in the breast, and localized lumps. Superficial lymphadenopathy may be involved, resulting in pain, suppuration, interference with breastfeeding, and inconvenience for daily life.

Tui na duration: 1 to 3 minutes for each technique.

Principles of treatment: To soothe the liver and clear heat, promote lactation, and reduce swelling.

Points to note: Wash nipples frequently with warm and soapy water to keep them clean, breastfeed regularly to prevent milk retention, treat nipple injuries promptly, and breastfeed only after the injuries heal.

Steps

❶ Pressing-kneading method: Stand behind the patient, and apply pressing-kneading on the Taiyang Bladder Meridian of Foot along both sides of the spine five times, focusing on the Ganshu, Pishu, and Weishu acupoints, until soreness is generated.

❷ Circular rubbing and pressing-kneading methods: Have the patient seated upright. Use the heel of the palm to apply circular rubbing, and three-finger pressing-kneading on the affected breast for 1 to 3 minutes. Keep the massage gentle, and then press-knead the Zhongwan, Tianshu, and Qihai acupoints with the finger.

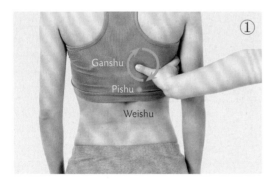

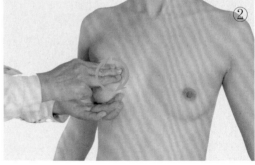

❸ Pushing method: Have the patient lying in supine position. Apply three-finger pushing from the armpits to the collar bone, then to the ribs and finally to the areola. Gradually increase the force applied and repeat 5 to 7 times for each part, milk can be seen flowing out while pushing.

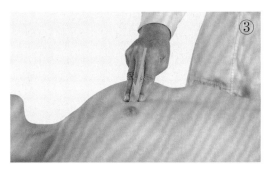
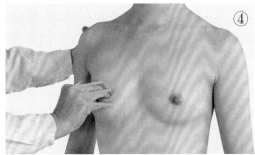

❹ Grasping method: Have the patient seated upright. Form a cupping shape with the tips of all fingers and prop up the nipple. Then gently grasp the areola 8 to 10 times with moderate strength. Note that at this point, a clotted grain-like blockage may be discharged with the milk.

❺ Pinching-grasping and plucking methods: Have the patient seated upright. Pinch-grasp the pectoralis major and latissimus dorsi muscles with five fingers, lifting and pinching before releasing. Then, apply the plucking method on the tendons with force, three times each.

❻ Pressing-kneading and twisting-rubbing methods: Have the patient seated upright. Press-knead the Danzhong acupoint with the index and middle fingers for one minute. Then, apply the twisting-rubbing method on both sides of the ribs for 3 to 5 minutes.

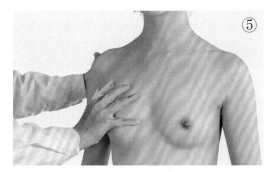
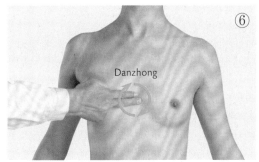

8. Mammary Gland Hyperplasia

Mammary gland hyperplasia refers to hyperplasia of the breast epithelium and fibrous tissue, structural degenerative lesions of the ducts and lobules of the breast tissue, and the growth of progressive connective tissue. Its cause is mainly an endocrine hormone imbalance. Mammary gland hyperplasia is a common breast condition in women, and should be prevented before it develops.

Liver depression and phlegm coagulation type mammary gland hyperplasia: Lumps and pain on one or both sides of the breast, related to the menstrual cycle. The lumps are small, slow to develop, not red or hot, can be moved by pushing, aggravated before menstruation, and alleviated after menstruation, accompanied by emotional disorders; irritability, insomnia and dreaminess, chest tightness and belching, chest pain, with a light tongue and thin white coating.

Thoroughfare-controlling vessels disharmony type mammary gland hyperplasia: Lumps and pain on one or both sides of the breast, lumps are larger, solid and hard, with heavy discomfort; often accompanied by irregular menstruation, reduced menstrual flow, light color discharge, or amenorrhea; accompanied by fear of cold, waist and knee weakness, fatigue, tinnitus, light fat tongue, thin white coating.

Basic Steps

❶ Kneading, circular rubbing, and pressing-kneading methods: Have the patient lying in supine position. Gently knead and rub the breast and the Rugen and Danzhong acupoints. Then, press-knead the Zhongwan, Tianshu, and Qihai acupoints for 1 to 2 minutes each. Next, knead and rub the stomach and abdominal area for 3 to 5 minutes until soreness is generated.

❷ Single finger meditation pushing and pressing-kneading methods: Have the patient lying in a prone position. Apply single finger meditation pushing along the Taiyang Bladder Meridian of Foot on the back repeatedly, then press-knead the Ganshu, Pishu, and Weishu acupoints with the thumb pulp for two minutes each, until soreness is generated.

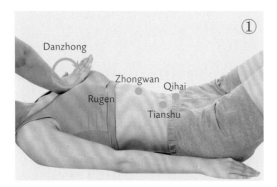
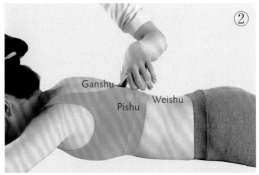

❸ Pressing-kneading method: Have the patient seated upright. Press-knead the Fengchi acupoint in a clockwise direction, then move down along the neck to the Dazhui acupoint. Press-knead 30 times back and forth along the way.

❹ Grasping-kneading method: Have the patient lying in a prone position. Grasp-knead the Jianjing acupoint for 3 to 5 minutes with all fingers, with moderate force.

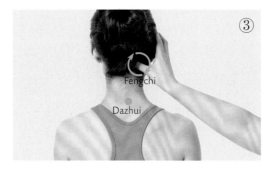
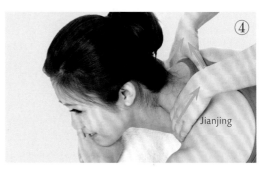

Additional Steps for Liver Depression and Phlegm Coagulation Type Mammary Gland Hyperplasia

❶ Kneading method: Have the patient seated upright. Knead the Yinlingquan acupoint with the thumb pulp for 1 to 3 minutes. More force can be applied.

❷ Kneading method: Have the patient seated upright. Knead the Ligou acupoint with the thumb pulp for 1 to 3 minutes with moderate force, until soreness is generated.

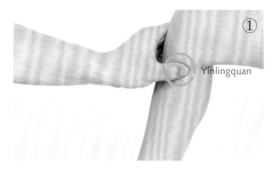
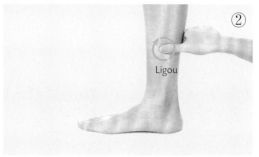

Additional Steps for Thoroughfare-Controlling Vessels Disharmony Type Mammary Gland Hyperplasia

❶ Pressing-kneading method: Press-knead the Shenshu acupoint with the thumb, then press-knead the Fenglong, Zusanli, and Sanyinjiao acupoints for 1 to 2 minutes each.

❷ To-and-fro rubbing method: Have the patient lying in a prone position. Stand on one side and rub the lumbosacral area transversely for 1 to 2 minutes until the heat generated penetrates the skin.

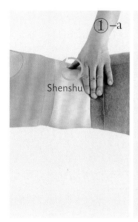
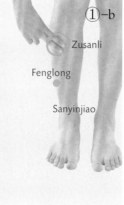
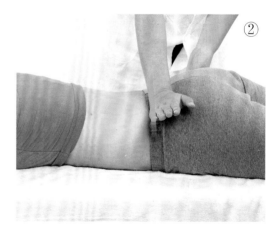

9. Prostatitis

Prostatitis, which belongs to the category of white turbidity in traditional Chinese medicine, is a common condition in middle-aged and elderly men. It is mainly caused by damp-heat diffusing downward and accumulate in the perineum. It is related to excessive alcohol consumption, perineal injury, and acute urethritis.

Tui na duration: 5 to 10 minutes for each body part.

Principles of treatment: To nourish the kidneys and benefit *qi*, strengthen the spleen to eliminate dampness, regulate *qi* and activate blood, clear heat and eliminate dampness.

Points to note: Take a warm bath in a seated position twice a day for 20 minutes each time, to help alleviate the symptoms.

Steps

❶ Pressing-kneading method: Have the patient lying in supine position. Stand on one side and apply the pressing-kneading method on the Qihai, Guanyuan, and Zhongji acupoints with the heel of the palm or the thumb pulp, for 5 to 10 minutes each. The force applied can gradually increase.

❷ Rolling method: Have the patient lying in a prone position. Apply the rolling method on their lumbosacral area for 5 to 10 minutes until the skin starts to feel warm.

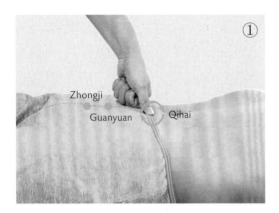
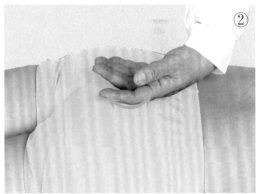

❸ Finger-pressing and kneading method: Have the patient standing. Finger-press and knead the Shenshu, Mingmen, Guanyuanshu, and Pangguangshu acupoints with the pulp of thumb or index finger for 5 to 10 minutes until soreness is generated.

❹ Finger pressing and to-and-fro rubbing methods: Have the patient lying in a prone position. Press the Baliao acupoints with the thumb pulp 50 times, then rub the palms against each other to generate heat before rubbing the Baliao acupoints until the heat generated penetrates the skin.

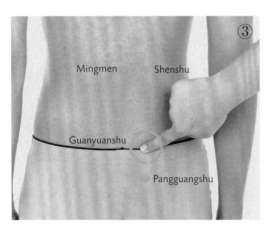
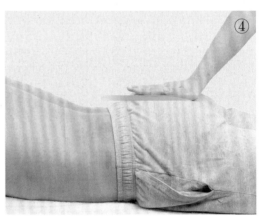

❺ Pinching-grasping method: Have the patient standing. Apply relative force on the thumb and index finger to pinch-grasp the Yinlingquan, Sanyinjiao, Taixi, Taichong and Dadun acupoints 30 to 50 times each.

❻ Pressing-kneading method: Have the patient sitting. Press-knead the Yongquan acupoint 100 to 200 times with the thumb pulp. Apply slightly more force, until soreness is generated.

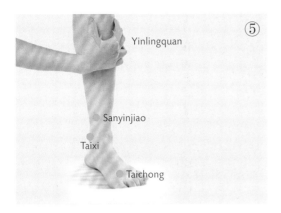

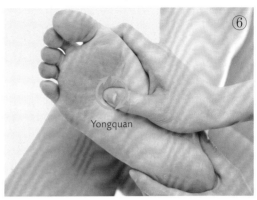

10. Impotence

Impotence is a condition in which an adult man's penis is either weak during sexual intercourse, or not hard, or is hard but for too short a duration to have a normal sex life. The external causes of this disease are mainly strain and injury, prolonged illness, poor diet, emotional problems, and external pathogens. The pathology include damage to the internal organs, *yin* and *yang* imbalance, block of *qi* and blood, or meridian obstruction, resulting in a lack of nourishment of penis and testes.

Tui na duration: 2 to 5 minutes for each body part.

Principles of treatment: To nourish the kidneys to revitalize potency.

Points to note: Eliminate burdensome thoughts, have a wide range of hobbies, and partake in social activities more regularly.

Steps

❶ Pressing-kneading method: Have the patient lying in a supine position. Press-knead the Shenque acupoint (navel) with the heel of the palm, until the part below the navel feels warm. The force applied should be gentle and deep, for 2 to 5 minutes.

❷ Kneading method: Have the patient lying in a supine position. Knead the Qihai, Guanyuan, and Zhongji acupoints with the thumb for two minutes each. Then, apply palm kneading on the Qihai and Guanyuan acupoints for 3 to 5 minutes, until soreness is generated.

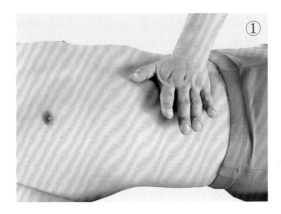

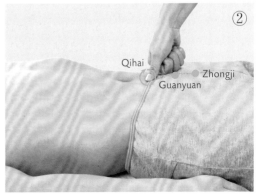

❸ Circular rubbing method: Have the patient lying in a supine position. Rub the abdomen area with the palm with gradually increasing force and amplitude, until a warm feeling is generated.

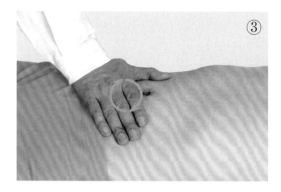

❹ Pressing-kneading method: Have the patient standing. Press-knead the Xinshu, Pishu, Shenshu, and Mingmen acupoints with the thumb or index finger. In addition, press-knead the Sanyinjiao acupoint on the lower limb. Massage with slightly more force for two minutes each, until the patient starts to experience a warm feeling on their stomach.

❺ Vibrating method: Have the patient lying in a prone position. Stand on one side and apply the vibrating method on the lower waist and lumbosacral area, until a warm feeling is generated.

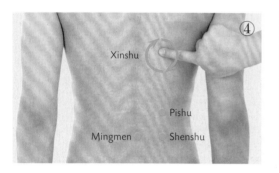

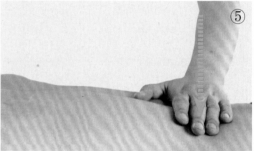

❻ To-and-fro rubbing method: Have the patient lying in a prone position. Stand on one side and apply the to-and-fro rubbing method with the hypothenar on the Yaoyangguan acupoint transversely until the heat generated penetrates the skin.

❼ Grasping method: Have the patient lying in a prone position. Grasp the inner thigh muscles with moderate force for two minutes.

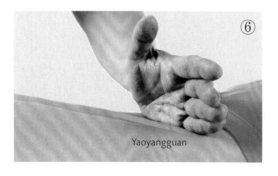

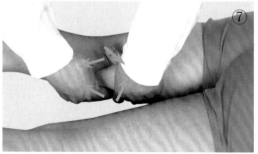

11. Premature Ejaculation

Premature ejaculation during intercourse is a condition that affects men's sexual life. It is a common condition of male sexual dysfunction, mostly accompanied by seminal emission and impotence. The most frequent causes of premature ejaculation are internal injury of emotions, dampness and heat attack, being too sexually active, and deficiency of the body due to prolonged illness.

Tui na duration: 3 to 5 minutes for each body part.

Principles of treatment: To nourish *yin* and lower fire, warm the kidneys and renew bodily essence, nourish the heart and spleen, consolidate astringency, and stop emissions.

Points to note: Participate in outdoor sport training to improve physical health.

Steps

❶ Pressing-kneading method: Have the patient lying in a supine position. Press-knead the Shenque acupoint (navel) with the heel of the palm, until the part below navel feels warm. The force applied should be deep and gentle, for 3 to 5 minutes.

❷ Kneading method: Have the patient lying in a supine position. Knead the Qihai, Guanyuan, and Zhongji acupoints with the thumb pulp for one minute each. Then, apply palm kneading on the Qihai and Guanyuan acupoints for 3 to 5 minutes.

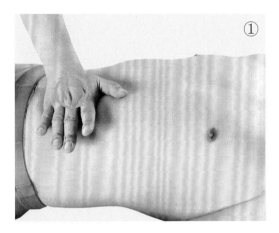

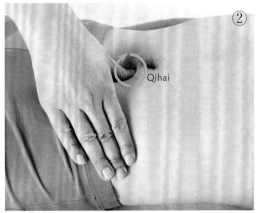

❸ Rolling method: Have the patient lying in a prone position. Apply the rolling method on the patient's lumbosacral area for 3 to 5 minutes. Keep the motion slow and the amplitude small.

❹ Finger-pressing and kneading method: Have the patient lying in a prone position. Press and knead the Shenshu acupoint with the thumb for 3 to 5 minutes until soreness is generated.

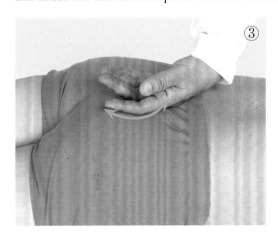

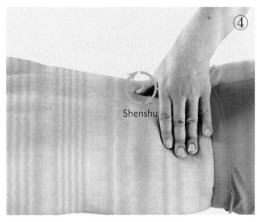

❺ Finger-pressing and kneading, pressing-kneading, and palm twisting methods: Have the patient lying in a prone position. Finger-press and knead the Baliao acupoints, and then press-knead the Baliao acupoints for 3 to 5 minutes. Apply palm twisting on the lower back until the heat generated penetrates the skin. (The patient should preferably be topless during the massage.)

❻ Grasping method: Have the patient lying in a prone position. Grasp the patient's inner thigh muscles with moderate force for two minutes.

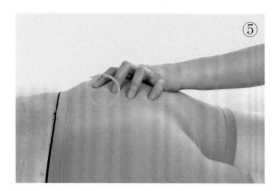
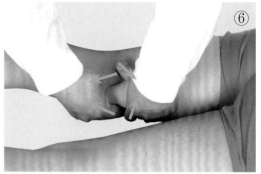

12. Seminal Emission

Seminal emission is ejaculation of semen without sexual intercourse or masturbation. It is normal for men to have some seminal emission during puberty. However, if it occurs too many times it is pathological, and is often related to neurasthenia or inflammation of the reproductive system.

Tui na duration: 3 to 5 minutes for each body part.

Principles of treatment: To nourish the kidneys and consolidate bodily essence.

Points to note: Adhere to a physical training regime to improve physical health. Maintain hygiene and keep good habits in daily life.

Steps

❶ Kneading and circular rubbing methods: Have the patient lying in supine position. Knead the Shenque acupoint with the heel of the palm until the patient feels warmth in the abdominal area. Then, apply circular rubbing on the lower abdomen for about five minutes.

❷ Finger-pressing and kneading method: Finger-press and knead the Xinshu, Ganshu, Danshu, Shenshu, Xiaochangshu, and Pangguangshu acupoints with the pulp of thumb or index finger for five minutes each.

❸ Rolling and to-and-fro rubbing methods: Have the patient lying in a

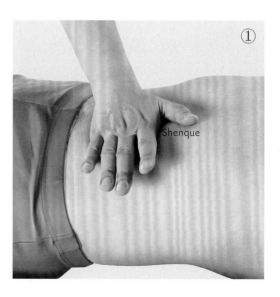

prone position. Roll the lumbosacral area for about three minutes, then rub the Mingmen, Shenshu, and Yaoyangguan acupoints, and the lumbosacral area transversely with gentle and even force until the heat generated penetrates the skin.

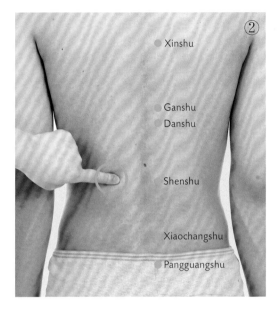

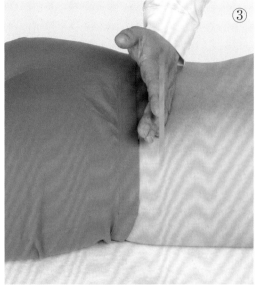

❹ Finger pressing method: Use the thumb pulp to press the Neiguan and Shenmen acupoints on the upper limb with a gradual increase in force.

❺ Pressing-kneading and rolling methods: Have the patient lying in a prone position. Press-knead the Sanyinjiao and Taixi acupoints with the thumb pulp for 1 to 2 minutes each, then roll the inner side of the lower limbs for 3 to 5 minutes.

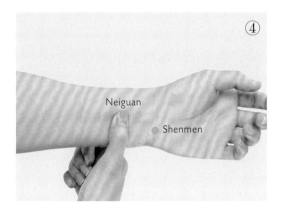

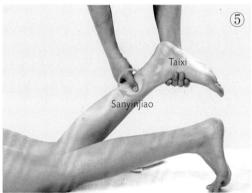

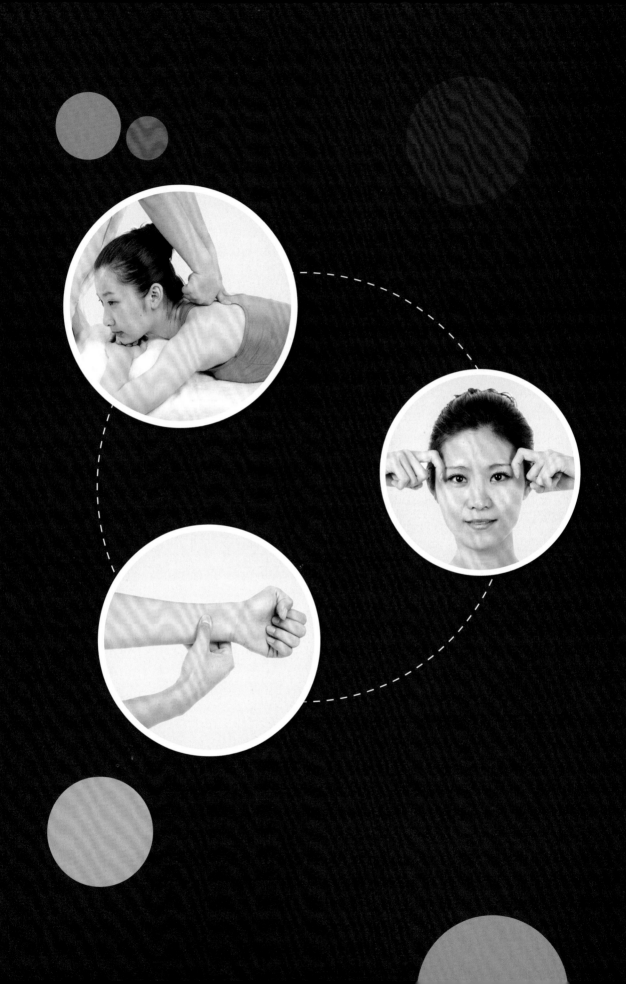

CHAPTER FIVE
Daily *Tui Na* to Improve Health

As well as alleviating illnesses, *tui na* massage has an effect on general health. This is because it can improve blood circulation, relieve fatigue, clear the brain, and freshen the mind. It also helps with aesthetic improvement. Performing *tui na* massage daily can enhance immunity, cure illnesses, and improve health.

Note: Some photographs in this book do not have acupoints marked out due to the angle at which they were taken. Please refer to the appendix for the list of commonly used acupoints in *tui na*. Massage both acupoints if they are symmetrically distributed on the body.

1. Head Care

Traditional Chinese medicine believes that the blood essence of internal organs and clear *yang qi* are gathered in the head. The head is susceptible to invasion from pathogenic *qi*. When people are exposed to a variety of internal and external pathogens, or after the completion of arduous work, they are likely to experience symptoms such as headaches, fatigue, and insomnia and lethargy. Therefore, ancient and modern healthcare methods focus on the health of the head, and a head massage is a good way to maintain it.

Tui na duration: Approximately two minutes for each body part.

Principles of treatment: To unblock the meridians and calm the nerves.

Points to note: Pay attention to resting and rest cycles. This will keep you energetic and clear-headed.

Steps

❶ Pushing method: Have the patient lying in a supine position. Stand on the right side or right behind their head. Push from the Yintang acupoint to the Shenting acupoint with alternating thumbs 30 to 50 times with moderate force.

❷ Pressing-kneading method: Have the patient seated upright. Press-knead the Baihui, Sishencong, and Touwei acupoints with the thumb pulp 30 to 50 times. Regular application of this massage helps to calm the nerves and keep the mind clear.

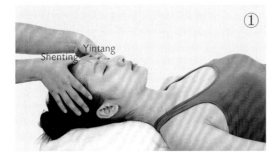
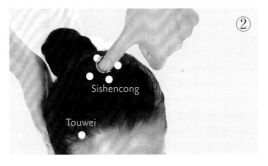

❸ Pushing method: Have the patient lying in a supine position. Use both palms to push from the forehead to the Taiyang acupoints on both sides. Then, push from the mastoid process area at the back auricle to the Fengchi acupoints. Repeat each action 3 to 5 times with slightly more force.

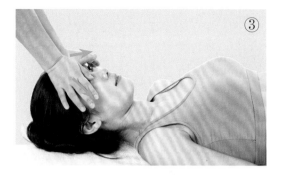

③

❹ Striking method: Cup both hands on the ears, with the heel of the palms facing forward and the fingers behind the head. Strike the back of the head three times with the index fingers, the middle fingers and the ring fingers, then quickly remove the hands from the ears. Repeat this nine times.

❺ Pinching-grasping method: Have the patient either standing up or seated. Pinch and grasp the Tianzhu, Fengchi, Fengfu, and Jingbailao acupoints forcefully 10 to 20 times. The force applied should be continuous, deep penetrating and ideally cause a strong sore feeling at various acupoints.

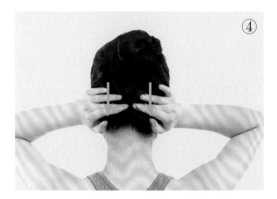

④

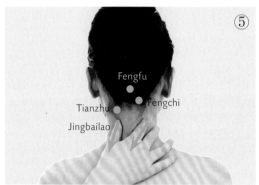

⑤

Fengfu
Fengchi
Tianzhu
Jingbailao

❻ Grasping and pinching-grasping methods: Have the patient standing. Grasp the head top with five fingers, move downwards and then use a three-finger grasp for the back of the head. Then, pinch and grasp the neck 3 to 5 times. This method should be continuous without any breaks in between.

❼ Grasping method: Have the patient standing. Grasp the head from above the ears with both hands. Apply the grasping method towards the side of the head 3 to 5 times. When executing this method, the fingers should exert relative force.

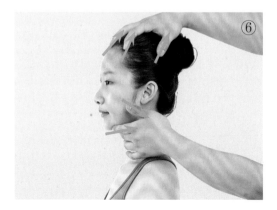

⑥

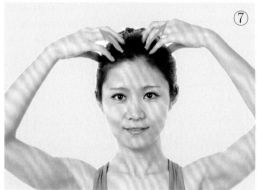

⑦

2. Eye Care

The eyes are the windows to the soul. Eye problems can cause great inconvenience for daily life. *Tui na* massage can keep our eyes healthy. Massaging the acupoints around the eyes can help dredge the meridians to reconcile *qi* and blood and eliminate eye muscle fatigue, so as to protect eyesight and prevent myopia.

Tui na duration: Approximately one minute for each body part.

Principles of treatment: To dredge the meridians and clear eyesight.

Points to note: Perform this routine once in the morning and evening and when the eyes feel fatigued.

Steps

❶ Pressing-kneading method: Place the pulp of both index fingers on each side of the Taiyang acupoint. Press-knead in both clockwise and anti-clockwise direction for one minute each, until soreness is generated.

❷ Pressing method: Place the pulp of index fingers on the Jingming acupoints and apply the pressing method downwards and upwards repeatedly until soreness is generated.

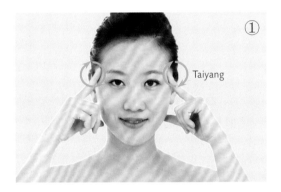
① Taiyang

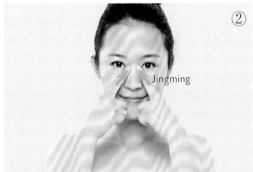
② Jingming

❸ Pressing-kneading method: Place the pulp of both index fingers on the Sibai acupoints and apply the pressing-kneading method. Pressing should be performed with slightly more force, and kneading should be kept gentle. Repeat until soreness is generated.

❹ Pressing-kneading method: Place the pulp of index fingers on the Chengqi acupoints and gently apply the pressing-kneading method. Keep the massage gentle to prevent injuring the skin.

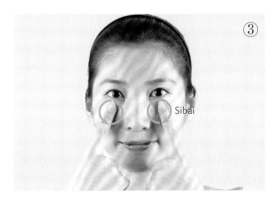
③ Sibai

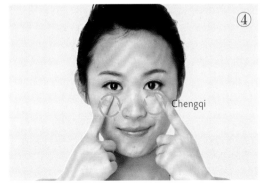
④ Chengqi

❺ Pushing-rubbing method: Flex and arch both index fingers and place them on the orbitals. Apply the pushing-rubbing method from the inside out, then top down repeatedly until soreness is generated.

❻ Pressing method: Press the Shangyang acupoint with the tip of the thumb, and gradually apply force until soreness is generated.

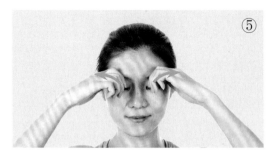

❼ Pressing-kneading method: Press-knead the Guangming acupoint with the thumb pulp for about one minute, with slightly more force, until soreness is generated.

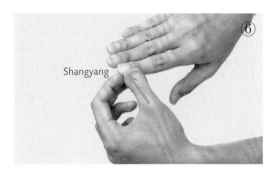

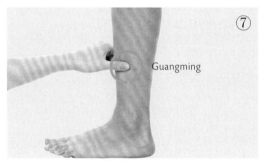

3. Face Care

Skincare is important to a lot of people. Apart from using skincare products, *tui na* massage is also a good way to maintain healthy skin. Regular *tui na* massage on the face can promote blood circulation, make the skin rosy and shiny, minimize facial wrinkles, and keep the face looking young. The following are some basic *tui na* techniques for facial care.

Tui na duration: Approximately one minute for each body part.

Principles of treatment: To promote *qi* and blood circulation, and to keep skin healthy.

Points to note: Warm the palms up by rubbing them against each other prior to commencing the *tui na* massage. Keep the force applied for the massage light.

Steps

❶ Pressing-kneading method: Press-knead the Touwei acupoint with the thumb pulp for 1 to 3 minutes daily. This helps to reduce crow's feet. This massage can be performed on

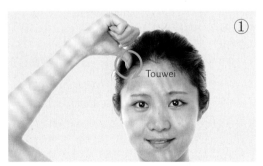

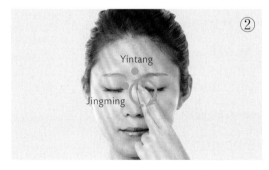

both sides simultaneously.

❷ Pressing-kneading method: Place the index finger on the middle finger and apply the pressing-kneading method on the Yintang and Jingming acupoints daily for one minute each, until soreness is generated. It can prevent wrinkles on the forehead and around the eyes.

❸ Pushing method: Have the patient lying in a supine position. Push with the thumb pulp from the Cuanzhu acupoint to the Taiyang acupoint. Repeat 5 to 8 times.

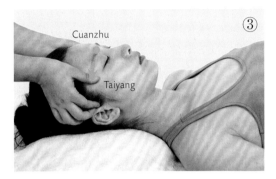

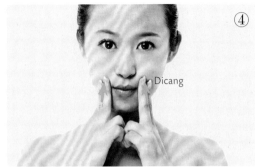

❹ Pressing method: Press the Dicang acupoints with the index and middle fingers. This can help minimize wrinkles around the mouth.

❺ Pressing method: Gently press the Quanliao acupoints with the middle and ring fingers from the bottom up 5 to 8 times. This helps to regulate the *qi* and blood in the face, keeping it moisturized and glowing.

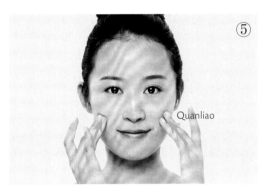

4. Chest and Abdominal Care

Strong internal organs ensure that the *qi* and blood are active, which in turn means a healthy body. Metabolism is the work of the internal organs, and functional internal organs are the foundation to a strong and healthy body. However, these organs are located deep in the chest and abdominal cavity, below the skin, muscles, and bones. Hence, applying *tui na* massage on the chest and abdominal is an easy way to maintain the health of our internal organs.

Tui na duration: 3 to 5 minutes for each body part.

Principles of treatment: To promote and regulate the flow of *qi* movement.

Points to note: A bare upper body during *tui na* session gives a better effect. Be mindful of keeping warm after the session.

Steps
❶ Single finger meditation pushing method: Have the patient lying in a supine position. Apply the single finger meditation pushing method on the Danzhong, Rugen, Shangwan, Zhongwan, Tianshu, and Qihai acupoints for three minutes each, until soreness is generated.

❷ Single finger meditation pushing method: Have the patient lying in a supine

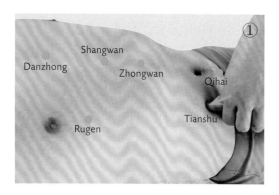

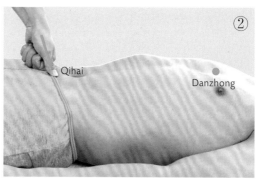

position. Apply the single finger meditation pushing method from the Qihai acupoint to the Danzhong acupoint. Repeat 2 to 3 times back and forth along the way.

❸ Pushing method: Have the patient lying in a supine position. Apply the pushing method from the Danzhong acupoint out towards the nipples. Repeat for 1 to 2 minutes.

❹ To-and-fro rubbing method: Have the patient lying in a supine position. Use the palm to rub transversely, from the collar bone downwards to the Danzhong, Rugen, and Jiuwei acupoints.

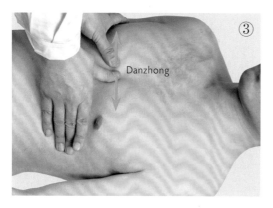

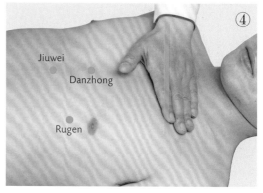

❺ Palm twisting method: Have the patient seated upright. Stand behind them and place both palms on each side of their ribs. Apply the palm twisting method with a gradual increase in force, until the skin is warm.

❻ Circular rubbing method: Have the patient seated upright. Apply the circular rubbing method with three fingers on the Danzhong acupoint for 1 to 3 minutes until the skin feels warm.

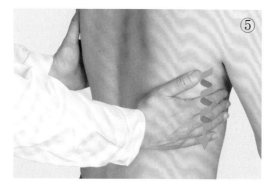

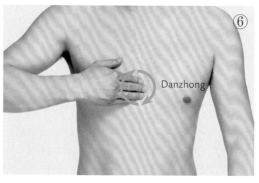

❼ Circular rubbing method: Have the patient lying in a supine position. Apply the circular rubbing method with three fingers or the palm on the Zhongwan, Tianshu, and Qihai acupoints for 3 to 5 minutes each. The force applied should start light and get heavier.

❽ Circular rubbing method: Have the patient lying in a supine position. Apply the circular rubbing method with the palm on the abdomen in a clockwise direction for five minutes.

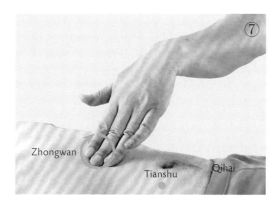

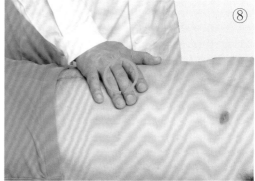

❾ Kneading method: Have the patient lying in a supine position. Knead the Tiantu, Danzhong, Zhongwan, and Shenque acupoints with the pulp of middle finger. Note that the force applied should be steady and even.

❿ Pressing method: Have the patient lying in a supine position. Press the Zhongwan, Qihai, and Guanyuan acupoints with the thumb. Note that the direction of force should be vertically downwards, and the force applied should gradually increase.

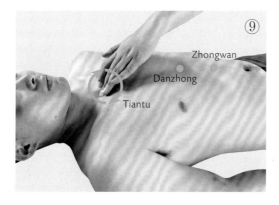

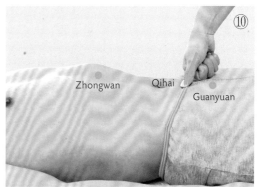

⓫ Vibrating method: Have the patient lying in a supine position. Place one hand on the patient's chest and abdominal area, and channel the force on the fingertips and palm. Strongly contract the forearm and hand muscles, so that the arm creates a strong vibration that is channeled through the fingertips and palm. Let the palm rest naturally on the patient, and do not apply additional force.

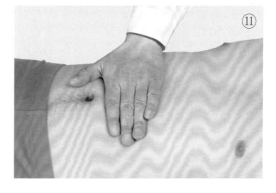

5. Back Care

Many adults have had experience with lower back pain, especially office workers who sit in front of a computer for long hours. The following are some *tui na* massage techniques for the back.

Tui na duration: 3 to 5 minutes for each body part.

Principles of treatment: To regulate and repair the tendons, dredge meridians, and activate collateral.

Points to note: Do not apply too much force during *tui na* massage, to prevent injuring the skin.

Steps

❶ Pushing and palm twisting methods: Rub the palms against each other to warm them up and place them on the waist. Push and palm twist the waist quickly in an up-and-down motion, so that the heat can penetrate to the deep tissues. This method should be executed quickly, increasing the area of treatment. The duration should ideally be 3 to 5 minutes.

❷ To-and-fro rubbing method: Place the hypothenar on the lower back and apply the to-and-fro rubbing method transversely. The force applied should be deep and slow, to allow the heat generated to penetrate deeply. The duration should ideally be three minutes.

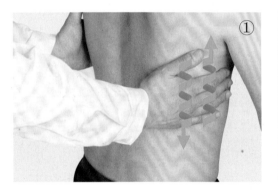
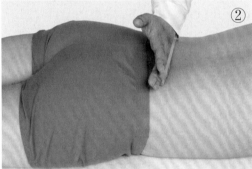

❸ Striking method: Clench both hands to form an empty fist and gently strike on the Shenshu and Mingmen acupoints with side of fist in alternate hands.

❹ Single finger meditation pushing method: Have the patient lying in a prone position. Apply the single finger meditation pushing method from the lower back to the Dazhui acupoint.

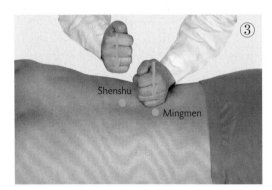
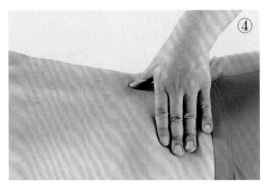

❺ Pushing method: Have the patient lying in a prone position. Apply the pushing method with the elbow on the Jiaji acupoints. Note that the force applied should be steady and the motion should be slow.

❻ Vibrating method: Have the patient lying in a prone position. Apply the vibrating method with the palm on the Mingmen and Yaoyanguan acupoints. The frequency of the vibrations should be high, ideally to allow the heat generated to penetrate the patient's skin.

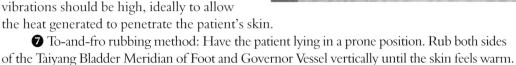

❼ To-and-fro rubbing method: Have the patient lying in a prone position. Rub both sides of the Taiyang Bladder Meridian of Foot and Governor Vessel vertically until the skin feels warm.

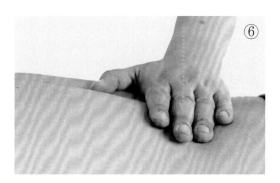
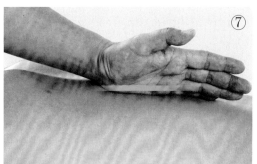

6. Limb Care

Limbs are vital body parts for mobility, and the body's vitality is correlated to their strength. Generally speaking, well-built and agile limbs are signs that the person is healthy and energetic; weak limbs and sluggish motion indicate that the person is weak. Hence, *tui na* massage for the limbs should be emphasized as part of a healthcare routine.

Tui na duration: 3 to 5 minutes for each body part.

Principles of treatment: To dredge meridians, activate collaterals, and lubricate the joints.

Points to note: This helps patients who are fatigued or experience sore limbs to alleviate their discomfort.

Steps

❶ Single finger meditation pushing method: Have the patient seated upright with their arms open. Apply the single finger meditation pushing method around the shoulder joint area for 3 to 5 minutes. Lubricant can be thinly applied to the treatment area before the massage.

❷ Single finger meditation pushing method: Apply the single finger meditation pushing method with the thumb pulp from the Jianyu acupoint towards the Quchi, Shousanli, and Hegu acupoints. Repeat 2 to 3 times back and forth along the way.

❸ Rolling method: Apply the rolling method with the back of the palm on the front of the shoulder joint. This massage can be supplemented with internal and external joint rotation. The amplitude of rolling should be moderate and kept steady.

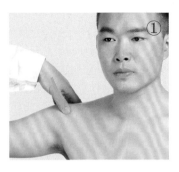
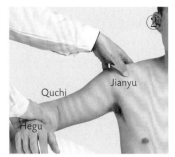
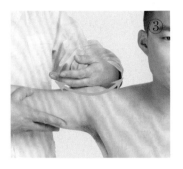

❹ Rolling method: Apply the rolling method on the back side of the patient's shoulder, ideally at a speed of 120 to 160 times per minute. This massage can be supplemented with joint stretches and internal rotations. Repeat 2 to 3 times.

❺ Pressing-kneading method: Use the pulp of index finger to press-knead the Jianliao, Jianzhen, and Tianzong acupoints in a clockwise direction until soreness is generated.

❻ Pressing-kneading method: Use the thumb pulp to press-knead the Quchi, Shousanli, Xiaohai, and Waiguan acupoints for 1 to 3 minutes each.

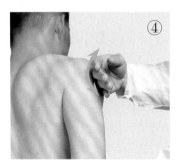
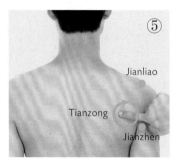
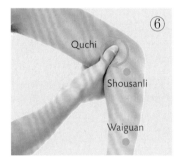

❼ Grasping method: Grasp the shoulder joint and the Jiquan and Shaohai acupoints with the thumb and other four fingers. The force applied should be moderate. Shake the shoulder joint after the massage.

❽ Stretching method: Stretch the shoulder joint, wrist joint, and finger joints. The force applied should gradually increase.

❾ Palm twisting method: Apply the palm twisting method with both palms on the shoulder joint and the upper limb 2 to 3 times. Repeat until the skin feels warm.

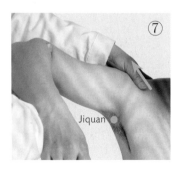
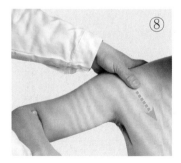
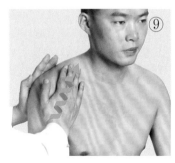

❿ Shaking method: Hold the patient's hand with both hands and shake the upper limb with a gradual increase in magnitude. The patient should not hold their breath during the massage.

⓫ Holding twisting method: Use the thumb and index finger to hold and twist the finger joints. Hold the fingers naturally without applying additional force.

⓬ To-and-fro rubbing method: Use the palm to rub on the shoulder joint, elbow joint, and wrist joint, until the skin feels warm.

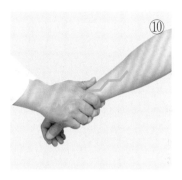
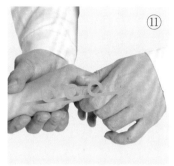
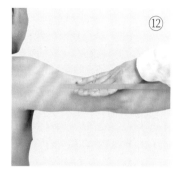

⓭ Rolling method: Apply the rolling method with the back of the palm along the Huantiao, Weizhong, and Chengshan acupoints 5 to 10 times. Roll from the groin to the adductor, quadriceps, knee, anterolateral calf, ankle, foot-back. Repeat 2 to 3 times back and forth on both legs. The movement should be steady and the technique should be soft.

⓮ Rotating method: Have the patient lying in a supine position with the knee bent at approximately 90°. Hold the patient's knee with one hand and the ankle with the other. Shake the hip, knee, and ankle joints. The movements should be slow, and the amplitude should not be too large.

⓯ Stretching method: Have the patient lying in a supine position. Prop up the patient's legs, and pull in the opposite direction to stretch the hip, knee, and ankle joints.

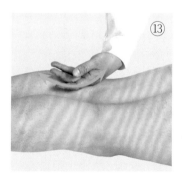
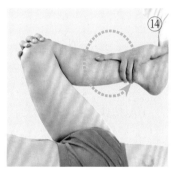
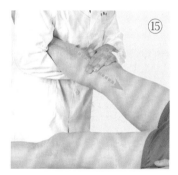

7. Lung Expansion and *Qi* Regulation

Applying *tui na* massage to the chest and abdomen can achieve lung expansion and *qi* regulation. With a good flow of *qi* in the chest, the heart and lungs can function optimally. Therefore, ailments such as chest tightness, wheezing, palpitations, and coughing can be prevented and treated with lung expansion and *qi* regulation.

Tui na duration: 3 to 5 minutes for each body part.

Principles of treatment: To condition and regulate *qi* movement.

Points to note: Maintain a positive mood.

Steps

❶ Pushing method: Push with both thumbs and thenars from the Conception Vessel located at the sternum to the sides of the chest, then push upwards to the collar bone.

❷ Circular rubbing and kneading methods: Use the palm or four fingers to perform circular rubbing, followed by kneading on the chest. If you are executing this with four fingers, place emphasis on the pectoralis major and pectoralis minor. This method should not be executed on an empty stomach. It should ideally be performed around half an hour after a meal.

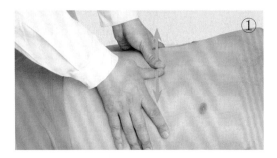 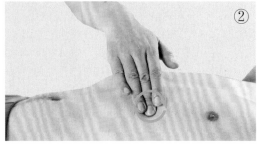

❸ Pressing method: Stack both palms together and press on the lower portion of the breastbone. The method should be executed slowly, in tandem with the breathing. Press down when the patient is breathing out, and release pressure when the patient is breathing in. Note that the palms should not be lifted from the patient.

❹ Kneading and pushing methods: Use four fingers to knead from the inside to the outside of the rib cage. Then, use thumb pulp to apply the pushing method from the inside to the outside of the rib cage.

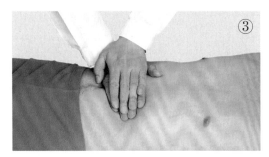 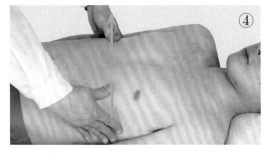

❺ Palm twisting method: Have the patient standing, and stand behind them. Place both palms on the side of the ribs and apply the palm twisting method, until the area feels warm.

❻ Finger pressing method: Use the thumb pulp to press on the Danzhong, Tianxi, Zhongfu, and Yunmen acupoints for 3 to 5 minutes each with moderate force.

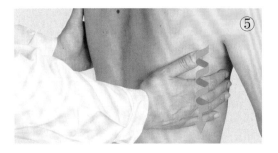 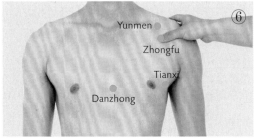

❼ Pushing method: Use both thumbs and thenars to push from the Conception Vessel to the sides of the ribs along the costal arch a few times, then push downwards towards the abdomen, starting respectively from the Shangwan, Zhongwan, and Shenque acupoints and push towards both sides. The force applied should be moderate.

❽ Circular rubbing method: Use the circular rubbing method with the palm from the umbilicus and move in the direction of intestinal peristalsis. Keep the force moderate and the speed slow. The duration of this method is slightly longer.

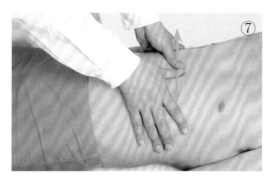
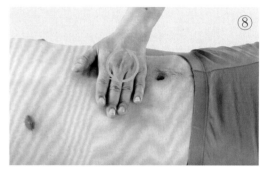

❾ Kneading method: Use the palm to knead the abdomen slowly with more force. Move in the direction of intestinal peristalsis. Knead on each area ten times before moving on to the next.

❿ Finger pressing and kneading methods: Use the index, middle, and ring fingers together to press the Xiawan, Tianshu, Qihai, Guanyuan, and Shuidao acupoints to dredge and regulate *qi* in the abdomen. If there is any area of pain, gently press and knead with your fingers for a while until soreness is generated.

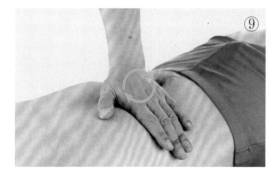
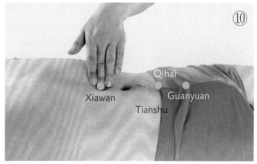

8. Invigorating the Stomach

In traditional Chinese medicine, the stomach is deemed as the foundation of acquired constitution, and the origin of *qi* and blood formation. Overeating or eating hard-to-digest food can increase the burden on the stomach, affecting normal digestive function. Therefore, it is beneficial to perform some *tui na* massage after a meal to help with digestion.

Tui na duration: Approximately three minutes for each body part.

Principles of treatment: To strengthen the spleen and stomach.

Points to note: Eat your meals on time, and keep the quantity moderate. Do not overeat or eat too little.

Steps

❶ Pressing-kneading method: Have the patient standing. Press-knead the Pishu, Weishu, and Dachangshu acupoints with the pulp of index finger to boost digestion.

❷ Pressing-kneading method: Have the patient lying in a supine position. Press-knead the Zhongwan acupoint with the palm with moderate force in a clockwise direction, for about three minutes. This helps to alleviate the bloated feeling after a meal.

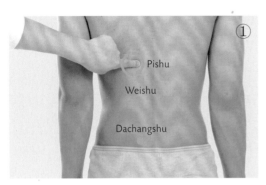
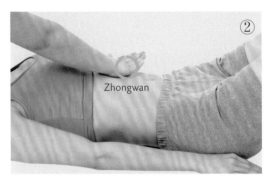

❸ Pressing and striking methods: Have the patient lying in a prone position. Press on both sides of the Dachangshu acupoints with the thumb pulp about 20 times. Use slightly more force. Alternatively, gently strike the Dachangshu acupoints with the fists about 20 times on each side.

❹ Pushing method: Have the patient lying in a supine position. Push downwards with slightly more force, with the heel of the palm from the Danzhong acupoint to the area around the Guanyuan acupoint. Repeat 3 to 6 times.

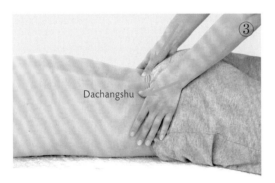
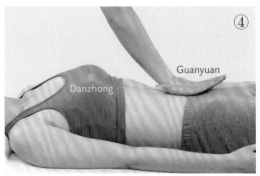

9. Calming the Heart and Tranquilizing the Mind

People nowadays are subjected to high stress at work and in life, and often suffer from insomnia and stress. These conditions can be alleviated with some *tui na* massage techniques. Below are some that you can perform regularly to calm your mind and maintain your mental health.

Tui na duration: Approximately three minutes for each body part.

Principles of treatment: To calm the heart and tranquilize the mind.

Points to note: Stay optimistic and keep your emotions stable.

Steps

❶ Pressing method: Have the patient seated upright. Press the Baihui acupoint with the pulp of the index finger. Gradually increase the force.

❷ Pressing method: Have the patient standing. Press the Shenshu acupoint firmly with the thumb pulp.

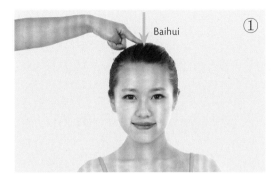

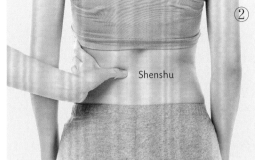

❸ Pressing and striking methods: Have the patient lying in a prone position. Press the Xinshu acupoint with the thumb pulp with a gradual increase in force. Alternatively, gently strike the same acupoint with a fist.

❹ Pressing method: Press the Neiguan acupoint with the thumb pulp 20 to 30 times. Keep the force steady and slow, until soreness is generated.

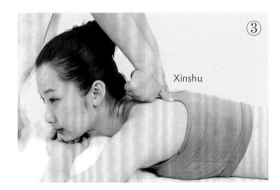

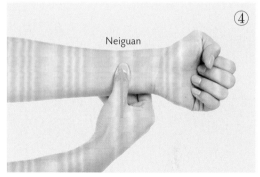

❺ Pinching method: Pinch the Shaoshang, Shaochong, and Laogong acupoints with the tips of the thumb and index finger for about one minute each, until soreness is generated.

❻ Pressing method: Have the patient seated upright. Press the Taixi acupoint with the thumb pulp until soreness is generated.

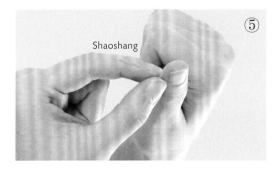

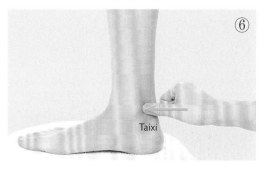

10. Soothing the Liver and Regulating *Qi*

Traditional Chinese medicine believes that the liver controls conveyance and dispersion and can regulate the *qi* within the body, which in turn promotes the function of internal organs and the circulation of *qi*, blood and body fluids. When a person's mood fluctuates, the functions of the liver can be affected, resulting in abnormalities in the *qi*'s activities, such as turbulent flow, stagnation, and reflux. Hence, it is important to learn *tui na* massage techniques that can help soothe the liver and regulate *qi*.

Tui na duration: Approximately 1 to 2 minutes for each acupoint.

Principles of treatment: To soothe the liver and regulate *qi*, to dredge the meridians, and activate collaterals.

Points to note: Manage your emotions, and remain happy and emotionally stable.

Steps

❶ Pushing and to-and-fro rubbing methods: Have the patient seated upright with both hands placed horizontally under the armpits. Keep the fingers open. The gap between each finger should be the same as the ribs. Push and to-and-fro rub towards the midline of the abdomen until the heat generated penetrates the skin.

❷ Kneading method: Have the patient seated upright. Place four fingers of either the left or right hand on the Danzhong acupoint and knead in a clockwise direction and an anti-clockwise direction with slightly more force for about one minute each way.

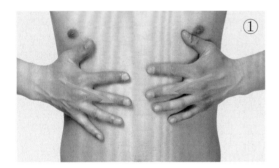
①

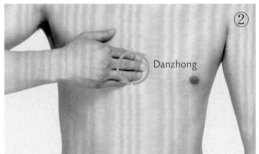
② Danzhong

❸ Pressing-kneading and plucking methods: Have the patient seated upright. Press the thumb on the Yanglingquan acupoint and use the other four fingers as support. Press-knead the acupoint for one minute, then pluck the tendon around the area transversely 3 to 5 times, until a sore, numb, and bloated feeling is generated.

❹ Pinching and kneading methods: Have the patient seated upright. Place the tip of the

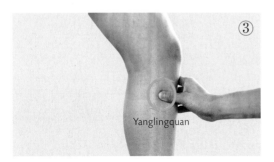
③ Yanglingquan

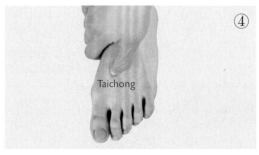
④ Taichong

thumb on the Taichong acupoint and apply pinching with slightly more force for about one minute. Then, place the thumb pulp on the acupoint and knead gently. Repeat for the other foot.

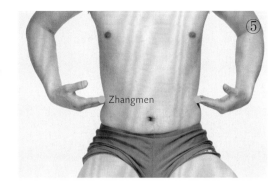

❺ Finger pressing method: Press both sides of the Zhangmen acupoint with the tip of the middle fingers for about one minute. Apply slightly more force, until a sore, numb, and bloated feeling is generated.

11. Slimming

As well as affecting the physical appearance, obesity also causes a variety of conditions such as high cholesterol, high blood pressure, coronary heart disease, cerebrovascular disease, and diabetes. These are "invisible killers" that threaten our health and lives. Therefore, losing weight is a pursuit of health and beauty to many people. The following *tui na* massage techniques can help with slimming to a certain extent, and are effective if performed long term.

Tui na duration: 1 to 2 minutes for each acupoint.

Principles of treatment: To dredge the meridians and activate collaterals.

Points to note: Keep your diet light, avoid greasy food and alcohol, have more fruit and vegetables, and consume appropriate amounts of protein. Maintain a diet that is low in fat, sugar, and salt.

Steps

❶ Sit-ups: Do 3 to 5 sets of sit-ups on the bed every day when you wake up or before you turn in. Each set should range between 8 to 12 repetitions. Do not do this exercise half an hour after eating.

❷ Abdominal breathing: Lie down in a supine position. Commence quick abdominal breathing to fill the abdomen up quickly. When exhaling, slowly lift your feet to 40° to 60°. Slowly put down your feet when you inhale. Repeat 20 to 30 times.

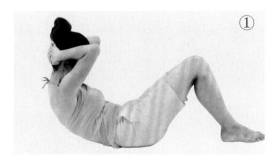

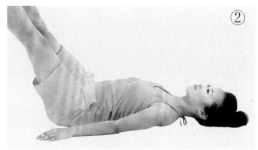

❸ Pressing-kneading method: Have the patient lying in a supine position. Press-knead the abdomen for 5 to 8 minutes with both palms. The force should gradually increase.

❹ Pinching and holding-twisting methods: Have the patient lying in a supine position. Pinch and lift the abdominal muscles with both hands 10 to 20 times. Apply the holding-twisting method on the muscles with the fingers after lifting. Hold 10 to 20 seconds before releasing slowly. Pinch with moderate force.

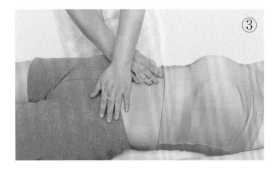
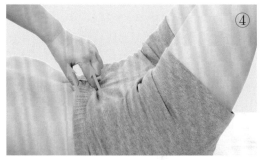

❺ Finger pressing method: Have the patient lying in a supine position. Press the Zhongwan, Qihai, and Tianshu acupoints with the thumb pulp for 5 to 8 minutes.

❻ To-and-fro rubbing method: Have the patient lying in a supine position. Rub the abdomen with the palm for five minutes until the skin feels warm.

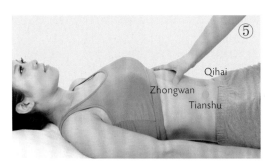
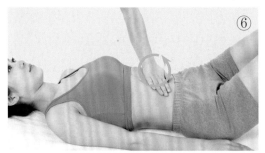

❼ Pressing-kneading method: Have the patient lying in a prone position. Press-knead along the Taiyang Bladder Meridian of Foot on both sides of the spine from the waist to the glutes 3 to 5 times, until soreness is generated.

❽ Pushing and to-and-fro rubbing methods: Have the patient lying in a prone position. Apply the to-and-fro rubbing method with palm heel on the waist before pushing to the glutes, until the heat generated penetrates the skin.

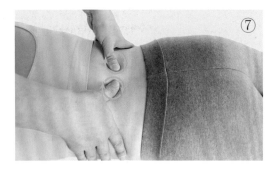
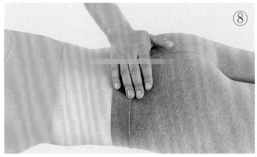

❾ Kneading-pinching method: Have the patient lying in a prone position and keeping the glutes relaxed. Knead, pinch, and lift the glute muscles with the fingers 10 to 20 times.

❿ Pressing method: Have the patient lying in a prone position. Press the Huantiao,

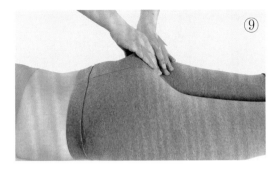

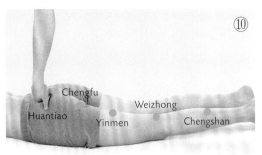

Chengfu, Yinmen, Weizhong, and Chengshan acupoints for 3 to 5 minutes each.

⓫ Pressing-kneading method: Have the patient lying in a supine position. Press-knead the Zusanli and Sanyinjiao acupoints on both legs for 3 to 5 minutes. The force applied should gradually increase, until local soreness is generated.

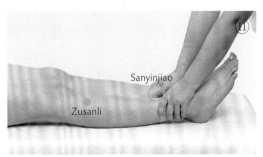

12. Improving Beauty

Tui na massage can also help to improve one's appearance. Applying *tui na* massage regularly on the acupoints on the face can help improve the blood circulation, help with absorption of nutrients through the capillaries and lymphatic tissues, expel metabolites, remove aging keratin, and increase the skin's elasticity, hence slowing down the aging of the skin.

Tui na duration: Approximately two minutes for each acupoint.

Principles of treatment: To improve the appearance.

Points to note: The *tui na* massage should ideally commence half an hour after a meal. One should not do this massage in a hungry or overfilling state.

Steps

❶ Pushing method: Place the thenars on the Yintang acupoint and have the heel of the palm firmly stuck on the superior margin of both eye sockets. Push outwards with slightly more force, towards the Taiyang acupoints 10 to 20 times.

❷ Pushing method: Place both thumbs on both sides of the Taiyang acupoints. Flex and

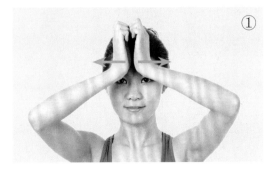

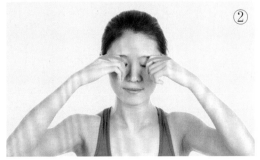

arch the index fingers and push from the Yintang acupoint outwards along the orbitals and gently push the eyelids.

❸ Pinching method: Pinch and lift the skin at the corner of the Taiyang acupoints with the second joint of the index fingers and the thumbs. Pinch and release 10 to 20 times.

❹ Pushing method: Slightly bend the index fingers and gently push from eyebrow arches to the Taiyang acupoints. Repeat 5 to 10 times.

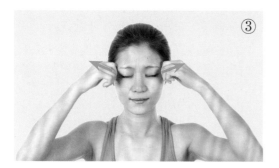
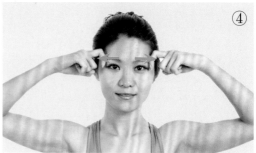

❺ Pushing method: Use the index and middle fingers to slowly push the lower eyelids on both sides upwards, then slowly push them back to the original position. Keep the force applied moderate and repeat 5 to 10 times.

❻ Pressing-kneading method: Use the thumb pulp to gently press-knead the Ermen, Tinggong, Tinghui and Yifeng acupoints.

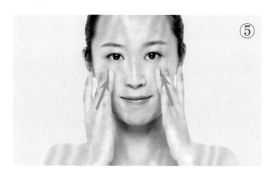
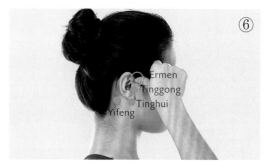

❼ Pressing-kneading method: Use the index and middle fingers together to press-knead the Dicang, Jiache, and Yingxiang acupoints for one minute each, until soreness is generated.

❽ Pressing-kneading method: Use the thumb pulp to press-knead the Chengjiang and Lianquan acupoints with moderate force until soreness is generated.

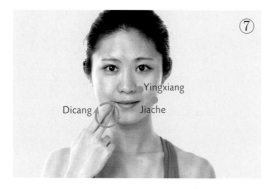
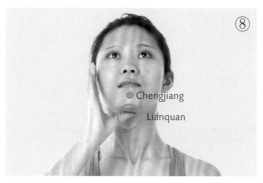

❾ To-and-fro rubbing method: Rub the palms against each other to generate heat, then press them onto the face and rub to-and-fro, as if you were washing it, until the entire face feels slightly warm.

❿ To-and-fro rubbing method: Lift the lower jaw and rub to-and-fro the neck for 10 to 20 times with one palm until the heat generated penetrates the skin.

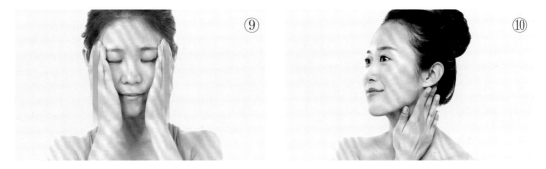

⓫ To-and-fro rubbing method: Use one palm to rub to-and-fro along the lower jaw 10 to 20 times until the heat generated penetrates through, then change to the other side of the jaw.

⓬ Pushing and to-and-fro rubbing methods: Use both index fingers to rub the sides of the nose bridge 10 to 20 times, until soreness and numbness is generated.

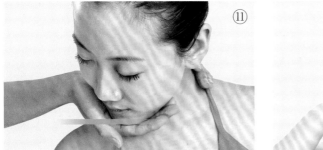

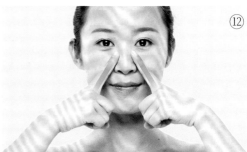

Commonly Used Acupoints in *Tui Na*

Acupoint	Location	Code
Baihui	On the head, 5 cun superior to the anterior hairline, on the anterior midline.	GV 20
Baliao	There are eight Baliao points in total, four on each side of the sacral spine. These are the upper, secondary, middle and lower Baliao points. They are located respectively in the first, second, third and fourth posterior sacral foramina (opening between vertebrae).	BL 31–34
Bingfeng	In the scapular region on both sides of the body, in the supraspinatous fossa, superior to the midpoint of the spine of the scapula.	SI 12
Changqiang	In the perineal region, inferior to the coccyx, midway between the tip of the coccyx and the anus.	GV 1
Chengfu	On both sides of the buttock region, at the midpoint of the gluteal crease.	BL 36
Chengjiang	On the face, in the depression in the center of the mentolabial sulcus.	CV 24
Chengqi	On both sides of the face, between the eyeball and the infraorbital margin, directly inferior to the pupil.	ST 1
Chengshan	On the posterior aspect of both legs, at the connecting point of the calcaneal tendon with the two muscle bellies of the gastrocnemius muscle.	BL 57
Chize	On the anterior aspect of both elbows, at the cubital crease, in the depression lateral to the biceps brachii tendon.	LU 5
Cuanzhu	On both sides of the head, in the depression at the medial end of the eyebrow.	BL 2
Dachangshu	On both sides of the lumbar region, at the same level as the inferior border of the spinous process of the fourth lumbar vertebra, 1.5 cun lateral to the posterior midline.	BL 25

Acupoint	Location	Code
Dadun	On the great toes of both feet, lateral to the distal phalanx, 0.1 cun proximal to the lateral corner of the toenail, at the intersection of the vertical line of the lateral side of the nail and the horizontal line of the toenail base.	LR 1
Daheng	On both sides of the upper abdomen, 4 cun lateral to the center of the umbilicus.	KI 12
Daimai	On the lateral abdomen, inferior to the free extremity of the 11th rib, at the same level as the center of umbilicus.	GB 26
Daling	On the anterior aspect of both wrists, between the tendons of palmaris longus and the flexor carpi radialis, on the palmar wrist crease.	PC 7
Danshu	On both sides of the upper back region, at the same level as the inferior border of the spinous process of the tenth thoracic vertebra (T 10), 1.5 cun lateral to the posterior midline.	BL 19
Danzhong	On the medial aspect of both feet, posteroinferior to the medial malleolus, superior to the calcaneus, in the depression anterior to medial attachment of the calcaneal tendon.	CV 17
Dazhu	On both sides of the upper back region, at the same level as the inferior border of the spinous process of the first thoracic vertebra (T 1), 1.5 cun lateral to the posterior midline.	BL 11
Dazhui	In the posterior region of the neck, in the depression inferior to the spinous process of the seventh cervical vertebra, on the posterior midline.	GV 14
Dicang	On both sides of the face, 0.4 cun lateral to the angle of the mouth.	ST 4
Dingchuan	On the spine area, at the same level as the inferior border of the spinous process of the seventh cervical vertebra, and 0.5 cun lateral to the middle line of the back.	EX-B 1
Dubi	On anterior aspect of both knees, in the depression lateral to the patellar ligament.	ST 35
Ermen	On both sides of the face, in the depression between the supratragic notch and the condylar process of the mandible.	TE 21
Feishu	In the upper back region, at the same level as the inferior border of the spinous process of the third thoracic vertebra, 1.5 cun lateral to the posterior midline.	BL 13

Acupoint	Location	Code
Fengchi	In the posterior region on both sides of the neck, inferior to the occipital bone, in the depression between the origins of sternocleidomastoid and the trapezius muscles.	GB 20
Fengfu	In the posterior region on both sides of the neck, directly inferior to the external occipital protuberance, in the depression between the trapezius muscle.	GV 16
Fenglong	On the anterolateral aspect of both legs, lateral border of the tibialis anterior muscle, 8 cun superior to the prominence of the external malleolus.	ST 40
Fengmen	On both sides of the upper back region, at the same level as the inferior border of the spinous process of the second thoracic vertebra (T 2), 1.5 cun lateral to the posterior midline.	BL 12
Fengshi	On the lateral aspect of both thighs, in the depression posterior to the iliotibial band where the tip of the middle finger rests, when standing up with the arm hanging alongside the thigh.	GB 31
Fujie	On both sides of the lower abdomen, 1.3 cun inferior to the center of the umbilicus, 4 cun lateral to the anterior midline.	SP 14
Ganshu	On both sides of the upper back region, at the same level as the inferior border of the spinous process of the ninth thoracic vertebra, 1.5 cun lateral to the posterior midline.	BL 18
Gaohuang	On both sides of the upper back region, at the same level as the inferior border of the spinous process of the fourth thoracic vertebra (T 4), 3 cun lateral to the posterior midline.	BL 43
Geshu	On both sides of the upper back region, at the same level as the inferior border of the spinous process of the seventh thoracic vertebra (T 7), 1.5 cun lateral to the posterior midline.	BL 17
Gongsun	On the medial aspect of both feet, anteroinferior to the base of the first metatarsal bone, at the border between the red and white flesh.	SP 4
Guangming	On the fibular aspect of both legs, anterior to the fibula, 5 cun proximal to the prominence of the lateral malleolus.	GB 37
Guanyuan	On the lower abdomen, 3 cun inferior to the center of the umbilicus, on the anterior midline.	CV 4
Guanyuanshu	On both sides of the lumbar region, at the same level as the inferior border of the spinous process of the fifth lumbar vertebra (L 5), 1.5 cun lateral to the posterior midline.	BL 26

Acupoint	Location	Code
Heding	In front of both knees, at the depression on top of the center point of the patellar bottom.	EX-LE 2
Hegu	On the dorsum of both hands, radial to the midpoint of the second metacarpal bone.	LI 4
Huantiao	On both sides of the buttock region, at the junction of the lateral one third and medial two thirds of the line connecting the prominence of the great trochanter with sacral hiatus.	GB 30
Jiache	On both sides of the face, one finger breadth (middle finger) anterosuperior to the angle of the mandible.	ST 6
Jiaji	On the spine area, on both sides of the spinous from the first thoracic to the fifth lumbar, 0.5 cun lateral to the middle line of the back. There are seventeen points each side.	EX-B 2
Jianjing	At the midpoint of the line connecting the spinous process of the seventh cervical vertebra with the lateral end of both acromia.	GB 21
Jianwaishu	On both sides of the upper back region, at the same level as the inferior border of the spinous process of the first thoracic vertebra (T 1), 3 cun lateral to the posterior midline.	SI 14
Jianyu	On both shoulder girdles, in the depression between the anterior end of the lateral border of the acromion and the greater tubercle of the humerus.	LI 15
Jianzhen	On both shoulder girdles, posteroinferior to the shoulder joint, 1 cun superior to the posterior axillary fold.	SI 9
Jianzhongshu	On both sides of the upper back region, at the same level as the inferior border of the spinous process of the seventh cervical vertebra (C 7), 2 cun lateral to the posterior midline.	SI 15
Jianliao	On both shoulder girdles, in the depression between the acromial angle and the greater tubercle of the humerus.	TE 14
Jiexi	On the anterior aspect of both ankles, in the depression at the center of the front surface of the ankle joint, between the tendons of extensor hallucis longus and extensor digitorum longus.	ST 41
Jingming	On both sides of the face, in the depression between the superomedial parts of the inner canthus of the eye and the medial wall of the orbit.	BL 1

Acupoint	Location	Code
Jiquan	In the axilla on both sides of the body, in the center of the axillary fossa, over the axillary artery.	HT 1
Jiuwei	On the upper abdomen, 1 cun inferior to the xiphisternal junction, on the anterior midline.	CV 15
Jueyinshu	On both sides of the upper back region, at the same level as the inferior border of the spinous process of the fourth thoracic vertebra (T 4), 1.5 cun lateral to the posterior midline.	BL 14
Juliao	Midpoint of the line connecting the anterior superior iliac spine and the prominence of the great trochanter on both sides of body.	GB 29
Kongzui	On the anterolateral aspect of both forearms, on the line connecting Chize point (LU 5) with Taiyuan point (LU 9), 7 cun superior to the palmar wrist crease.	LU 6
Kunlun	On the posterolateral aspect of both ankles, in the depression between the prominence of the lateral malleolus and the calcaneal tendon.	BL 60
Laogong	On palm of both hands, in the depression between the second and third metacarpal bones, proximal to the metacarpophalangeal joints.	PC 8
Liangmen	On both sides of the upper abdomen, 4 cun superior to the center of the umbilicus, 2 cun lateral to the anterior midline.	ST 21
Liangqiu	On the anterolateral aspect of both thighs, between the vastus lateralis muscle and the lateral border of the rectus femoris tendon, 2 cun superior to the base of the patella.	ST 34
Lianquan	In the anterior region of the neck, superior to thyroid cartilage, in the depression superior to the hyoid bone, on the anterior midline.	CV 23
Lieque	On the radial aspect of both forearms, between the tendons of the abductor pollicis longus and the extensor pollicis brevis muscles, in the groove for the abductor pollicis longus tendon, 1.5 cun superior to the palmar wrist crease.	LU 7
Ligou	On the anteromedial aspect of both legs, at the center of the medial border (surface) of the tibia, 5 cun proximal to the prominence of the medial malleolus.	LR 5
Mingmen	In the lumbar region, in the depression inferior to the spinous process of the second lumbar vertebra (L 2), on the posterior midline.	GV 4

Acupoint	Location	Code
Neiguan	On the anterior aspect of both forearms, between the tendons of the palmaris longus and the flexor carpi radialis, 2 cun proximal to the palmar wrist crease.	PC 6
Neixiyan	On both knees, in the center of the depression of the patellar ligament.	EX-LE 4
Pangguangshu	In the sacral region, at the same level as the second posterior sacral foramen, and 1.5 cun lateral to the median sacral crest.	BL 28
Pishu	On both sides of the upper back region, at the same level as the inferior border of the spinous process of the 11th thoracic vertebra (T 11), 1.5 cun lateral to the posterior midline.	BL 20
Pucan	On the lateral aspect of both feet, distal to Kunlun point, lateral to the calcaneus, at the border between the red and white flesh.	BL 61
Qiaogong	The Qiaogong acupoint is located on both sides of the large tendon. It starts from the Yifeng acupoint behind the ears (in the depression between the front underside of the mastoid process and the lower jaw), along the straight line diagonally along the sternocleidomastoid muscle to the Quepen acupoint (which is located on the upper clavicle fossa).	/
Qihai	On the lower abdomen, 1.5 cun inferior to the center of the umbilicus, on the anterior midline.	CV 6
Qihaishu	On both sides of the lumbar region, at the same level as the inferior border of the spinous process of the third lumbar vertebra (L 3), 1.5 cun lateral to the posterior midline.	BL 24
Qihu	In the anterior thoracic region on both sides of the body, inferior to the clavicle, 4 cun lateral to the anterior midline.	ST 13
Qimen	On both sides of the anterior thoracic region, in the sixth intercostal space, 4 cun lateral to the anterior midline.	LR 14
Qiuxu	On the anterolateral aspect of both ankles, in the depression lateral to the extensor digitorum longus tendon, anterior and distal to the lateral malleolus.	GB 40
Quanliao	On both sides of the face, inferior to the zygomatic bone, in the depression directly inferior to the outer canthus of the eye.	SI 18
Quchi	On the lateral aspect of both elbows, at the midpoint of the line connecting Chize point (LU 5) with the lateral epicondyle of the humerus.	LI 11

Acupoint	Location	Code
Quepen	In the anterior region of the neck on both sides of the body, in the greater supraclavicular fossa, 4 cun lateral to the anterior midline, in the depression superior to the clavicle.	ST 12
Ququan	On the medial aspect of both knees, in the depression medial to the tendons of the semitendinosus and the semimembranosus muscles, at the medial end of the popliteal crease.	LR 8
Quze	On the anterior aspect of both elbows, at the cubital crease, in the depression medial to the biceps brachii tendon.	PC 3
Ran'gu	On the medial aspect of both feet, inferior to the tuberosity of the navicular bone, at the border between the red and white flesh.	KI 2
Rugen	On both sides of the anterior thoracic region, in the fifth intercostal space, 4 cun lateral to the anterior midline.	ST 18
Sanjiaoshu	On both sides of the lumbar region, at the same level as the inferior border of the spinous process of the first lumbar vertebra (L 1), 1.5 cun lateral to the posterior midline.	SL 22
Sanyinjiao	On the tibial aspect of both legs, posterior to the medial border of the tibia, 3 cun superior to the prominence of the medial malleolus.	SP 6
Shangjuxu	On the anterior aspect of both legs, on the line connecting Dubi point (ST 35) with Jiexi point (ST 41), 6 cun inferior to Dubi point (ST 35).	ST 37
Shangwan	On the upper abdomen, 5 cun superior to the center of the umbilicus, on the anterior midline.	CV 13
Shangxing	On the head, 1 cun superior to the anterior hairline, on the anterior midline.	GV 23
Shangyang	On the index finger of both hands, radial to the distal phalanx, 0.1 cun proximal-lateral to the radial corner of the index fingernail, at the intersection of the vertical line of the radial border of the fingernail and the horizontal line of the base of the index fingernail.	LI 1
Shaochong	On the little finger of both hands, radial to the distal phalanx, 0.1 cun proximal-lateral to the radial corner of the little fingernail, at the intersection of the vertical line of the radial border of the nail and horizontal line of the base of the little fingernail.	HT 9

Acupoint	Location	Code
Shaohai	On the anteromedial aspect of both elbows, just anterior to the medial epicondyle of the humerus, at the same level as the cubital crease.	HT 3
Shaoshang	On the thumb of both hands, radial to the distal phalanx, 0.1 cun proximal-lateral to the radial corner of the thumb nail, at the intersection of the vertical line of the radial border and the horizontal line of the base of the thumb nail.	LU 11
Shenmen	On the anteromedial aspect of both wrists, radial to the flexor carpi ulnaris tendon, on the palmar wrist crease.	HT 7
Shenque	On the upper abdomen, in the center of the umbilicus.	CV 8
Shenshu	On both sides of the lumbar region, at the same level as the inferior border of the spinous process of the second lumbar vertebra (L 2), 1.5 cun lateral to the posterior midline.	BL 23
Shenting	On the head, 0.5 cun superior to the anterior hairline, on the anterior midline.	GV 24
Shenzhu	On both sides of the upper back region, in the depression inferior to the spinous process of the third thoracic vertebra (T 3), on the posterior midline.	GV 12
Shidou	On both sides of the anterior thoracic region, in the fifth intercostal space, 6 cun lateral to the anterior midline.	SP 17
Shousanli	On the posterolateral aspect of both forearms, on the line connecting Yangxi point (LI 5) with Quchi point (LI 11), 2 cun inferior to the cubital crease.	LI 13
Shuidao	On both sides of the lower abdomen, 3 cun inferior to the center of the umbilicus, 2 cun lateral to the anterior midline.	ST 28
Sibai	On both sides of the face, in the infraorbital foramen.	ST 2
Sishencong	A group of four points, at the vertex, 1 cun respectively posterior, anterior and lateral to Baihui point.	EX-HN 1
Taichong	On the dorsum of both feet, between the first and second metatarsal bones, in the depression distal to the junction of the bases of the two bones, over the dorsalis pedis artery.	LR 3
Taixi	On the posteromedial aspect of both ankles, in the depression between the prominence of the medial malleolus and the calcaneal tendon.	KI 3

Acupoint	Location	Code
Taiyang	On both temples, between the tip of the brow and outer canthal, the depression that 1 cun behind and inferior to it.	EX-HN 5
Taiyuan	On the anterolateral aspect of both wrists, between the radial styloid process and the scaphoid bone, in the depression ulnar to the abductor pollicis longus tendon.	LU 9
Tianjing	On the posterior aspect of both elbows, in the depression 1 cun proximal to the prominence of the olecranon.	TE 10
Tianshu	On both sides of the abdomen, 2 cun lateral to the center of the umbilicus.	ST 25
Tiantu	In the anterior region of the neck, in the center of the suprasternal fossa, on the anterior midline.	CV 22
Tianxi	On both sides of the anterior thoracic region, in the fourth intercostal space, 6 cun lateral to the anterior midline.	SP 18
Tianzhu	In the posterior region on both sides of the neck, at the same level as the superior border of the spinous process of the second cervical vertebra (C 2), in the depression lateral to the trapezius muscle.	BL 10
Tianzong	In the scapular region on both sides of the body, in the depression between the upper one third and lower two thirds of the line connecting the midpoint of the spine of the scapula with the inferior angle of the scapula.	SI 11
Tinggong	On both sides of the face, in the depression between the anterior border of the center of the tragus and the posterior border of the condylar process of the mandible.	SI 19
Tinghui	On both sides of the face, in the depression between the intertragic notch and the condylar process of the mandible.	GB 2
Touwei	On both sides of the head, 0.5 cun directly superior to the anterior hairline at the corner of the forehead, 4.5 cun lateral to the anterior midline.	ST 8
Waiguan	On the posterior aspect of both forearms, 2 cun proximal to the dorsal wrist crease, midpoint of the interosseous space between the radius and the ulna.	TE 5
Waixiyan	Same as Dubi acupoint.	ST 35

Acupoint	Location	Code
Wan'gu	On the posteromedial aspect of both wrists, in the depression between the base of the fifth metacarpal bone and the triquetrum bone, at the border between the red and white flesh.	SI 4
Weishu	On both sides of the upper back region, at the same level as the inferior border of the spinous process of the 12th thoracic vertebra (T 12), 1.5 cun lateral to the posterior midline.	BL 21
Weizhong	On the posterior aspect of both knees, at the midpoint of the popliteal crease.	BL 40
Wuyi	On both sides of the anterior thoracic region, in the second intercostal space, 4 cun lateral to the anterior midline.	ST 15
Xiaguan	On both sides of the face, in the depression between the midpoint of the inferior border of the zygomatic arch and the mandibular notch.	ST 7
Xiajuxu	On the anterior aspect of both legs, on the line connecting Dubi point (ST 35) with Jiexi point (ST 41), 9 cun inferior to Dubi point (ST 35).	ST 39
Xiaochangshu	On both sides of the sacral region, at the same level as the first posterior sacral foramen, and 1.5 cun lateral to the median sacral crest.	BL 27
Xiaohai	On the posteromedial aspect of both elbows, in the depression between the olecranon and the medial epicondyle of the humerus bone.	SI 8
Xiawan	On the upper abdomen, 2 cun superior to the center of the umbilicus, on the anterior midline.	CV 10
Xingjian	On the dorsum of both feet, between the first and second toes, proximal to the web margin, at the border between the red and white flesh.	LR 2
Xinshu	On both sides of the upper back region, at the same level as the inferior border of the spinous process of the fifth thoracic vertebra (T 5), 1.5 cun lateral to the posterior midline.	BL 15
Xuanshu	In the lumbar region, in the depression inferior to the spinous process of the first lumbar vertebra (L 1), on the posterior midline.	GV 5
Xuanzhong	On the fibular aspect of both legs, anterior to the fibula, 3 cun proximal to the prominence of the lateral malleolus.	GB 39

Acupoint	Location	Code
Xuehai	On the anteromedial aspect of both thighs, on the bulge of the vastus medialis muscle, 2 cun superior to the medial end of the base of the patella.	SP 10
Yangchi	On the posterior aspect of both wrists, on the dorsal wrist crease, in the depression ulnar to the extensor digitorum tendon.	TE 4
Yangjiao	On the fibular aspect of both legs, posterior to the fibula, 7 cun proximal to the prominence of the lateral malleolus.	GB 35
Yanglingquan	On the fibular aspect of both legs, in the depression anterior and distal to the head of the fibula.	GB 34
Yangxi	On the posterolateral aspect of both wrists, at the radial side of the dorsal wrist crease, distal to the radial styloid process, in the depression of the anatomical snuffbox.	LI 5
Yaoshu	In the sacral region, at the sacral hiatus, on the posterior midline.	GV 2
Yaoyangguan	In the lumbar region, in the depression inferior to the spinous process of the fourth lumbar vertebra, on the posterior midline.	GV 3
Yifeng	In the anterior region of the neck, posterior to both ear lobes, in the depression anterior to the inferior end of the mastoid process.	EX-HN 14
Yinbai	On the great toe of both feet, medial to the distal phalanx, 0.1 cun proximal-medial to the medial corner of the toenail, at the intersection of the vertical line of the medial border and horizontal line of the base of the toenail.	SP 1
Yingxiang	On both sides of the face, in the nasolabial sulcus, at the same level as the midpoint of lateral border of the wing of the nose.	LI 20
Yinlingquan	On the tibial aspect of both legs, in the depression between the inferior border of the medial condyle of the tibia and the medial border of the tibia.	SP 9
Yinmen	On the posterior aspect of both thighs, between the biceps femoris and the semitendinosus muscle, 6 cun inferior to the gluteal fold.	BL 37
Yintang	The midpoint of the line between two eyebrows.	GV 29

Acupoint	Location	Code
Yongquan	On the sole of both feet, in the deepest depression when the foot is in plantar flexion.	KI 1
Yuji	On both palms, radial to the midpoint of the first metacarpal bone, at the border between the red and white flesh.	LU 10
Yunmen	On both sides of the anterior thoracic region, in the depression of the infraclavicular fossa, medial to the coracoid process of the scapula, 6 cun lateral to the anterior median line.	LU 2
Yuyao	On both sides of the forehead, superior to the pupil, at the midpoint of the eyebrow.	EX-HN 4
Zhangmen	On both sides of the lateral abdomen, inferior to the free extremity of the 11th rib.	LR 13
Zhaohai	On the medial aspect of both feet, 1 cun inferior to the prominence of the medial malleolus, in the depression inferior to the medial malleolus.	KI 6
Zhibian	In the buttock region, at the same level as the fourth posterior sacral foramen, 3 cun lateral to the median sacral crest.	BL 54
Zhishi	On both sides of the lumbar region, at the same level as the inferior border of the spinous process of the second lumbar vertebra (L 2), 3 cun lateral to the posterior midline.	BL 52
Zhiyang	In the upper back region, in the depression inferior to the spinous process of the seventh thoracic vertebra (T 7), on the posterior midline.	GV 9
Zhongfu	On both sides of the anterior thoracic region, at the same level as the first intercostal space, lateral to the infraclavicular fossa, 6 cun lateral to the anterior median line.	LU 1
Zhongji	On the lower abdomen, 4 cun inferior to the center of the umbilicus, on the anterior midline.	CV 3
Zhongwan	On the upper abdomen, 4 cun superior to the center of the umbilicus, on the anterior midline.	CV 12
Zusanli	On the anterior aspect of both legs, on the line connecting Dubi point (ST 35) with Jiexi point (ST 41), 3 cun inferior to Dubi point (ST 35).	ST 36